D0014747

Helene –
Love you, my sister.
Keep shining that beautiful
light!
Perfect Health

The Good Fight

Donna Hicken

Closet Books
Jacksonville

Copyright ©2004 by Donna Hicken

All rights reserved under International and Pan-American
Copyright Conventions. No part of this book may be
reproduced in whole or in part in any manner without written
permission of the publisher. Published in the United States by
Closet Books, a division of Robert Crane Publishing.

Closet Books and the book colophon are trademarks
of The Robert Crane Corporation. All other trademarks
marked or unmarked are property of their respective owners.

Dust jacket design by Joseph Schlosser
Cover photo courtesy Paul King
Back cover photo courtesy Donna Hicken

1st Edition

ISBN 1-891-23218-5

This book is in no way a representation of Medical fact or Medical
Procedure. It is for information only, and should not be considered
as medical advice. Please consult with your health practitioner
before considering any therapy or therapy protocol.

TM

Closet Books
PO Box 440504
Jacksonville, FL 32222

www.ClosetBooks.com

Printed in the United States of America
46809753

For Danielle and Drew

Contents

FOREWORD

They didn't train me for this in college. Some challenges were to be expected when I made the jump from the frontlines of journalism to management. Along the way, I was forced to do budgets, schedules and the other things that come with being the News Director of a local television station. Still, I was not prepared for the conversation Donna and I had to have.

Donna Hicken anchors the news in Jacksonville, Florida. In the most technical sense, I am her boss. Most would tell you we are co-workers. I call her my friend. It is in all these roles that I listened as she broke the news; she had breast cancer.

This was the first of two conversations. You see Donna has battled cancer twice. Before you move ahead into the tale of the second battle, I think you need some background on her first fight.

Our television station is known for our coverage of breast cancer. One of Donna's co-anchors and friend, Jeannie Blaylock, developed a program to encourage women to do self-breast exams each month. For nearly 10 years, on the 12th of every month (we work for Channel 12), Jeannie has done stories about women discovering lumps in their breasts through self-exams. Donna was doing a check when she discovered the original lump. The irony was not lost on any of us.

I always believed Donna would beat the cancer the first time. Don't get me wrong, I was worried and I cried when Donna and Jeannie saw each other for the first time after doctors delivered the news. Still, I expected her to continue to show up late for work, fight for more political coverage and run marathons for years to come. I didn't know what my role was supposed to be during this fight. I just knew Donna would win.

In the role as her boss, I had to convince Donna she had to tell her viewers about the cancer. It's tough being such a public person. You don't get to pick and choose when you are public and when you are private. Still, it felt like I was kicking her when she was down when I started the conversation. Donna didn't want to make a circus of her cancer. "No cameras at the treatments! No weekly updates." Donna was angry. I knew the cancer didn't stand a chance.

The conversation a few months later was much easier. Donna was preparing to take her last chemotherapy treatment. It was amazing. In a few short months, she had lost her hair, lost weight and lost the anger. She was bright-eyed and ready to move on with her life. Donna took a camera to the last treatment. She took her wig off and talked about the longest marathon of her life. She was a real winner that day!

That's what makes the second time we had the cancer conversation that much more difficult. When Donna looked at me with tears in her eyes and strain on her face, I knew this was not going to be the same fight the second time.

As one of our public service projects, the television station was building a Habitat for Humanity house when Donna learned she was heading back to chemo. Despite the devastating news and days of crying, Donna came out to the house to help build. She was in no shape to help her co-anchors lay sod. Donna and I took a walk. It was a beautiful late April Friday. We sat in a driveway a block down from the house we were building. Donna told me she didn't think she could do it again. She told me she did not have the strength to fight again. For the first time, I was not sure Donna was going to make it.

I have never told Donna about my thoughts after that conversation. For the first time, I had to think about how the newsroom would cope if Donna died. How would we cover it? How would I deal with the loss of one of my key people and close friends. I couldn't share those thoughts with her then; she could not take it.

Donna needed help to keep her focused on this final fight. Those are the seeds that led to Donna's Journal. Four years of college and a year of graduate work, prepared me to pick lead stories, ask tough questions and push for the truth. However, once again, I found myself sitting across from Donna talking about how we were going to keep her viewers informed about what she was going through. Donna agreed to write for our website once a week.

In our new cyber world, something wonderful started happening. Words of encouragement started flowing into the station. Like a crowd along the route of a marathon, the city of Jacksonville encouraged Donna to pick up her feet and power forward. The second half of this race, was much tougher than the first. Donna's body had not yet fully recovered from the first fight when they started pumping the poison called chemo back into her body. She was so sick, she would sometimes stay in the bathroom throwing up until minutes before air. She had so little energy, I wasn't sure she would be able to last for an entire newscast. Every time I encouraged her to take time off she said "No!" Donna barely missed a day during her eight month fight. The wonderful words that beamed in daily helped her continue down the track.

The saying goes, "It takes a village to raise a child." In this case, it took an entire community to conquer cancer. For years, Donna's undying spirit helped lift people across the First Coast. In the end, they gave back to help lift her. Donna refused to quit. She still attacks her job with a tremendous will to win. She attacks her personal life with the same winning will. It's a tremendous formula for life. They didn't teach me that in college; I learned it here.

J. Michael McCormick
News Director
First Coast News
WJXX-TV ABC 25 / WTLV-TV NBC 12

The Good Fight

Donna Hicken

INTRODUCTION

1 Timothy 1:18-19

"Timothy, my son, I give you this instruction in keeping with the prophecies once made about you, so that by following them you may fight the good fight, holding on to faith and a good conscience."

From the time I was a little girl, I knew I wanted to be a writer. I started writing my first book when I was in fifth grade, but I never had the attention span to finish.

Turns out I'm a deadline kind of girl. Give me too much time and I procrastinate.

Journalism was a perfect fit.

I never thought in a million years that breast cancer, my own at that, would be the impetus to write that long forgotten book.

But then, I never planned on Lynn Skapyak Harlin.

I'll never forget our first conversation. My former colleague Marcia Ladendorff e-mailed me and said she had a very talented writer friend who wanted to talk with me about doing a book. I was fairly certain this was insane, but at Marcia's urging I followed through.

I met Lynn on her shanty boat, docked at the Trout River near downtown Jacksonville. The boat is her refuge, and a place where she holds periodic writing seminars. She is, as Marcia described precisely, "a hoot."

Turns out, Lynn was in bed with her husband Jim, when she got the inspiration for the book. No, not that kind of inspiration.

She was actually watching me on TV. I was talking about my newly formed Foundation offering financial assistance to local women with breast cancer, when she sat straight up and proclaimed, "Oh damn!"

"What is it?" Jim asked.

I get the feeling Jim has been on the receiving end of Lynn's *eureka's* before.

"I have to help Donna Hicken write her book!" she answered, as if Jim was missing something obvious.

"What book?"

"Her book for the Foundation! Oh and I don't have time for that!"

"Then don't do it."

"I have to do it," she said. "She needs me."

Lynn and I talked for hours that first day.

I learned her inspiration actually came from personal experience. Lynn's godmother, Evelyn Pinneker, is fighting breast cancer. Evelyn lives in Nebraska, and Lynn can't be there to help. When Lynn saw me on TV that night, she knew instantly this was her way to make a difference.

As the senior editor for Closet Books, Lynn told me if I wrote a book about my on-line journal and my cancer experience, the company would donate all the net proceeds to the Donna Hicken Foundation!

I wrote the first chapter that night.

But you need to know this book isn't just about me. It's about the people who touched my life during my struggle with breast cancer and how we helped each other. It's a love story really. The best kind of love story.

As my husband is fond of saying, "We're all connected." I've never believed that more.

Acknowledgments

I want to thank you, Lynn, from the bottom of my heart for your guidance, your nagging, your commitment to excellence, your nagging, your friendship, and of course more nagging. You had the vision for this project from the start and it is your belief in it that made me believe. You've done your godmother proud.

George Gilpatrick, publisher of Closet Books, I forgive you for what Lynn put me through and I thank you as well for your incredible generosity.

Some wonderful writers donated their time and talent to tell the personal stories of the other survivors in this book. Katrina Mims-Cook, Amy Copeland, Oscar Senn, Bridget Willis Spruill, Dan Ovshak and Tonn Pastore. You are all awesome!

My special thanks to my friend, Julie Gillespie who correctly predicted she would do the lion's share of work to make The Donna Hicken Foundation a success. Julie, I told you on my 40th birthday, I'd get back at you for showing pictures of me (ON THE AIR!) in those hideous yellow bell bottoms from eighth grade.

To all of my DHF board members and other friends and family who will no doubt be embarrassed in some way in this book my thanks and my apologies.

To my First Coast News family: thanks for carrying me during my chemo when I couldn't carry myself, and for supporting this book wholeheartedly.

To Jeanette Ghiotto, and the folks from Catholic Charities, who partner with the Foundation, you walk the walk every day. Your example and dedication have been invaluable.

To the men, women and children who made Donna's Journal a beautiful path to healing, "Thank you" could never be enough.

To Elizabeth Hazouri, my mom, who taught me that there's truly no cure for a Catholic upbringing, I love you anyway.

To Donald Hazouri, my late father, who believed without a

doubt that I could do anything in the world, I miss you every moment.

To Tim Deegan, my husband, who agreed to let our life in a fishbowl become our life in a fishbowl under a magnifying glass, thank you for laughing and crying and living with me through these pages.

To Danielle and Drew, my children, I am grateful for every day I can watch you grow into the incredible people you are becoming. And I pray that in your lifetime, cancer will simply become a word in the medical history books.

You make it possible for me to fight the good fight.

ONE

A Simple Blood Test

It was a simple blood test. As if any blood test for a cancer patient could ever be simple. I had noticed the trend. My "marker," the test that tells me if I need to worry, had been up slightly for the past two years. First 40, then 45, 48, now 55.

But there was always a reason. All of my other blood work was normal, so my doctor wasn't worried. Except for that trend thing. She decided, just to be sure, to give me a PET scan. The state of the art in cancer detection.

Sitting in the waiting area, numb with fear, I had this feeling. I'd had it for a while. Physically, I felt fine. But the numbers bothered me. Why couldn't they just be NORMAL?

My doctor explained to me that five percent of women tested sit at the high end of "normal" or just above.

"That's a lot of women," she said.

I thought "Sure, I'm supposed to feel good that five percent is a lot of women, but I'm also supposed to feel good that I only have a 20 percent chance of getting cancer again. If five percent is high, why is 20 percent low?"

Such are the mind games of the cancer patient.

Staring at my fiancé, trying my best not to cry, I kept thinking, "OK, Donna, keep it together, everyone's watching you. Be cool, it's probably nothing." But my heart was racing and I couldn't stop the tears. I had come such a long way. I was finally where I belonged. Tim had asked me to marry him in October and we planned an August wedding.

I was sure this spelled my doom. Too happy, must be time for something bad to happen.

"Stop it!" I said aloud to fend off my thoughts.

All I wanted to do was escape my body. Be somewhere, anywhere else.

The nurse gave me an injection. Radioactive glucose. If I had cancer, I was told, it would beam like a light bulb when they scanned my body.

I was dressed in a white terry cloth robe, and placed in a long tube-like machine up to my forehead. The scan started at my feet and worked slowly upward. It took almost an hour. I can't honestly tell you what my thoughts were during that time. I was just surviving.

Looking at the scan would have been incredibly fascinating if it wasn't my own body.

A 3-D spinning me, rotating on the screen. Completely clear.

With the exception of one big beaming spot well above my right breast.

"So doc, could this be something else, something other than cancer?"

My voice was coming from someone else's body.

The doctor, a man I'd never seen, had his back to me facing the screen. I'm not sure I ever saw his face.

"It's possible, but not likely," he explained.

"A severely torn muscle perhaps," he continued, "but it would have to be very recent."

My head was playing a vicious game of tit-for-tat with my heart.

"OK," I'm thinking, "I did work out pretty hard yesterday. I even boxed. I'm awfully sore. Maybe."

There it is Donna. You see it. Get a grip.

"This can't be! I had a small tumor, they took it out, my lymph nodes were clean, chemo as an insurance policy! It was supposed to be a slam dunk!"

Calm down, compose yourself, you can deal with this.

The rest of that day and the next I felt like Gumby. Formless. Limp. Pulled from one place to the next. A CT scan, bone scan,

2

liver scan. Warm dyes pushing through my veins, lighting up every part of my body. A biopsy of "the mass" to determine once and for all what I was dreading.

My head was working overtime. *I can't do this again. I can't. I can't.*

*   *   *

I should have known this drama was coming when Cheryl Hesse showed up. She was down visiting from her home in Buffalo. Cheryl and I became friends when we were both living in West Palm Beach in 1987.

Shortly after I moved home to Jacksonville in '88, she moved back to Buffalo. Or as she says, "BEE-yak" to Buffalo. I love to tease her about her accent.

Cheryl has managed to show up for every major crisis of my life, and although quite unintentional, this was no exception. This was supposed to be a fun reunion. In fact our friend Jon Frankel was flying in from New York and we had planned a dinner at my favorite oceanfront restaurant, First Street Grille. I was determined to go ahead with it.

Tim and Cheryl chatted at the table. I sat staring at our sun-soaked view of the ocean, willing the peaceful scene to calm my brain when Jon showed up.

"Howya doin' Hicken?"

The familiar voice momentarily shattered my self pity.

"I'm peachy, Frankel, just peachy," I said sarcastically, reaching up to hug his neck.

Jon is a reporter for CBS news. He's got a face that turns heads, and a mind that keeps you there. He is also a first class smart ass. (My favorite feature).

Jon was a cub reporter during those days in West Palm, while I was a "seasoned" anchor of three years. We used to sit in the edit bays into the wee hours of the morning, cutting each other to the quick, carefully crafting resume tapes so that Jon could make his

3

escape to Miami, the next stepping stone.

He was a sports guy then, but we both knew he'd end up in news. His goal was always to get to New York where he grew up. Of course that also happens to be the top television market in the country. I never had a doubt he'd make it.

Jon was in Jacksonville for a follow up to the Brenton Bulter case. An African-American teen wrongly accused of murdering a white tourist. The story grabbed national headlines.

"Nice timing on the visit," I chided. "Always in the right place at the right time for bad news."

"I'm so sorry Donna. You OK, kiddo?" Jon's voice was soft, sympathetic.

Not you too, Jon.

Everyone was treating me like a victim. I needed my smart- ass friend to make me feel like me. Our relationship was based on mutual grief-giving. I wanted a return volley I could slam.

"Geez Frankel... Don't YOU pity me. You start being nice to me and I know I'm dead," I snapped playfully.

Jon half laughed, and lowered himself into a chair. Cheryl shot me an uneasy look.

"Tell me about your interview Jon," I said quickly, shifting to a well-worn path. "You talked with Shorstein, right?"

To my relief, Jon launched into a vintage Frankel description of our State Attorney.

"Tell me THAT guy doesn't have a high opinion of himself," he said loudly. "What an ego!"

An instant chorus of giggles came from the table next to ours.

"State Attorney's office," I whispered back at him.

Jon's face flushed.

We all lost it laughing.

"Thee-yats good, Frankel," Cheryl teased, "tee-yactful as usual."

It was the first time Tim and I had really laughed since the whole ordeal began. A much needed, if short, break from the mental grind. Two days wasn't long enough. I hated to see my friends go.

For the next several days I was in mourning. Someone had

4

died. I was still clinging to the tiniest hope that life as I knew it, wanted it, would continue.

"OK Lord, whatever you want," I'd say. As a nearly lifelong Catholic I have never felt comfortable praying for any particular outcome, just God's will for me.

"But you know Lord, if it IS what you want…. Oh God, please let it be what you want. Let me be all right," I was secretly begging.

In my calmer conversations with Him I would shake my head at my obsession with Catholic form.

As if there's a thought in my head You don't know.

By the end of all the poking and prodding, which covered the better part of a week, Tim and I walked into the Mayo Clinic to hear the sentence.

"I can't stand the smell here," I told him. Just entering the large double glass doors from the garage made me queasy. "I guess I just connect the smell to the whole experience. The needles, the nausea, the disease."

We sat in Dr. Edith A. Perez' office waiting for what seemed like an eternity. Edith is highly respected, the breast cancer director for the Mayo Clinic. She is from Puerto Rico, and small like me, with short dark wiry hair, and large brown eyes. She's often either totally absorbed in numbers or smiling like she's up to something. It is impossible not to like her.

Edith had become more than my doctor through all this, she was a good friend. And I knew she took this as personally as I did. I could tell she was miserable. We had both taken the attitude that we were done with this thing the first time. "Don't spend your time looking back," she would tell me. "People do that and they forget to live."

At the moment, I couldn't do much of either. I felt paralyzed.

Two taps on the door and Edith walked in.

" Donna, the cancer is back," she said, closing the door behind her. It was as if she just wanted to get the words out of her mouth quickly and let them evaporate into space.

After the PET scan the initial worry was that the cancer might

5

have metastasized, so I was literally holding my breath.

"Here is what I believe has happened," she said in her familiar formal Puerto Rican accent. She pulled out her pen, as she almost always did, to help me understand through illustrations. Edith is one of those rare doctors who seems to relish explaining the intricacies to her patients. At least to those who want to know. To me it says, "I care. You are not a number."

Elbows propped up on the table, she began to draw.

"This is your sentinel node. I believe that a cell or two from your original tumor went here. Cancer cells can hide in lymph nodes. They can be dormant during chemotherapy and then become active again."

"But I thought we removed my nodes and they were clean?"

"Those were your axillary nodes. This is a sentinel node. It is routinely tested now, but at the time, that was not the case. The good news here is that I believe this is not a new occurrence, but has been here all the time. Your liver, and other organs all look fine. OK?" She managed a smile and looked up from the paper to see that I understood.

The elephant eased off my chest. I nodded.

"Well, that's a huge Amen!" Tim said brightly.

"Absolutely," Edith agreed. "The lymph node is partly cancerous and partly normal. It will have to come out and you will have to have a new round of radiation and chemotherapy. I'm sorry, Donna."

And I knew she was, from the bottom of her heart.

It's truly amazing how fast the brain compensates. That survival instinct. I think I know in some small part what it's like to be a POW. Panic, resist, resign, assess, adjust to a new reality. Survive.

By the end of that exhausting day in Edith's office, Gumby was regaining her form. Yes, I would have to go through radiation again, chemo again, lose my hair again, puke again, feel like death again. But my doctor was relieved and optimistic about my prognosis.

"We are going to take care of it this time. We are going to be aggressive. I am not one to simply keep this at bay. I want it gone for good."

I was soon to find out exactly what she meant by *aggressive*. For now, I was just pleased I still had a life to plan. I squeezed Tim's hand.

"So," I said to him, "how do you feel about bald girls?"

"You know I'm just strange enough to like that," he grinned.

Thank God. If we were going to keep our August wedding date, my head would probably be as shiny as my ring by then.

My first phone call after I knew was to my mother.

I got all my worry genes from her and, true to character, she had already been around the beads about 30 times heading for rosary number 31 when she picked up the phone. My mother is as Catholic as it gets. The author, I believe, of Catholic guilt and self-recrimination. Not to mention far and away THE most dramatic person I've ever known. Having said that, she is also my rock in faith. When I was little I asked her if she was older than God.

"I assure you I am not," she answered in mock dismay. "God has always existed."

"Are you sure?" I persisted.

"Yes, Mooey, (her pet name for me) I'm absolutely sure," she said, smiling down her cheeks at me.

I have never doubted her.

"Mom, it's back."

"OH DAMN!" She began to cry. But before she could get herself into full throttle Elizabeth Hazouri hysteria…

"It's going to be OK," I said steadily.

Here I was comforting my mother. Explaining the plan. And it made me feel better. We do that for each other, in addition to driving each other the worst kind of crazy.

I'm used to the drill with my mom. It's weird, but there's a comfort zone there.

I felt no such comfort as I contemplated telling my children that my cancer had returned.

7

My sweethearts were so little the first time. Danielle was just seven when I was first diagnosed. Drew, five. I would have rather lit myself on fire than tell them I had cancer.

Now, two and a half years after that initial diagnosis, here we were again. I found myself fighting the conventional wisdom all the books had to offer. "Don't give children more information than they need. Children just need to feel secure."

Well, how the heck do I make them feel secure when I've got to tell them AGAIN that I have a life threatening disease?

"Mommy is going to be fine," I said, as they both sat blinking at me from their perch on the side of Danielle's bed. "I'll be tired again, and there will be some stuff I can't do for a while, but the doctors just need to give me more medicine to get rid of the cancer once and for all."

Danielle was examining my tear-swollen face.

"Why did it come back?"

"The doctors think they just didn't quite get all of it the first time," I said. "This time they will give me new, better medicine and then, hopefully, it will be gone for good."

"Does this mean you're going to be bald again?" Drew said, fighting a smile. My son, like me, smiles when he's uncomfortable.

"They aren't sure, Drewdy, but probably."

Danielle was embarrassed the first time I showed up without my wig or hat to pick her up from school. Drew thought it was flat out cool, even if it did scare him a little. Drew doesn't hesitate to tell me when something scares him. We even have in-depth talks about fearing death. Danielle, most of the time, keeps those thoughts to herself. She also has the worry gene. But she would never admit it to anyone. She is the kindest, most considerate person I know.

They took what I told them in stride, at least to my face. I would be fine. The alternative was not a place I could allow my mind to go. The thought of leaving them would leave me inconsolable.

After breaking the news to the rest of the family I turned to my other family, the viewers. By now I had come up off the mat and was back in the fight with fists flying. But I worried how the folks at home would handle this. I hated bringing it back to them. They'd been so good to me the first time. People must get sick of this stuff. I mean who wants to be reminded of their own mortality every day? They would once again have to see me wither, struggle for energy. I truly felt bad about that, and selfishly, I just didn't want to deal with the whole public thing all over again.

A cancer patient learns quickly that what you want doesn't matter squat. You do what you have to do. Period.

"So how do you want to do this?" My boss had a tough time meeting my eyes.

Mike is a tough cookie. He knows his stuff, and has a reputation as a hot head. Since I'm never one to back down from a good fight, we sometimes go at it like brother and sister. But as such, we are family.

Mike leaned over his desk. "Sometimes I don't know how you do it," he said, his eyes starting to well with tears. "I just look at you and you're so healthy. You exercise and you eat the right things. I can't stand that this is happening to you."

I was touched by his emotion, but I saw fear in his eyes and it scared me. I didn't linger there.

"I'm going to tape a statement for the viewers to be run the day I have my surgery," I said. "And I'm going to make jokes, like I always do. It helps me."

"OK, it's not the way I would handle it, but you have to be you."

Mike and I made a bet the first time I was diagnosed. He thought I couldn't get through telling the viewers without crying. "Bet I can," I said.

That night, live on the air, I told everyone I had cancer and then quipped, "And for those of you who are always complaining about my hairdo, good news. We'll get to start all over." I then blew a kiss to the camera, smiled, went to the end-break, and bawled my eyes out. But not on TV.

The day I went in for my surgery, my colleagues Jeannie

9

Blaylock and Alan Gionet anchored from the set, while my taped statement played for my viewers during the evening broadcast. "I'll be back with you tomorrow," I said. "Besides…Jeannie and Alan couldn't live without me."

The surgery had been scheduled hastily. Dr. William Fulmer was going to remove the cancer. I met with him after my pre-op tests.

"The lymph node we have to remove is very close to a major vein, Donna," he counseled. "I can't tell by looking at your ultrasound, but it may actually touch the vein. Not a good place to have cancer. That vein would provide easy transportation for those cells." Time was of the essence.

Dr. Fulmer shot from the hip. But there was something very warm and comforting in his manner. A confidence that wasn't at all cocky, but very reassuring. He was easy to talk with. His smile was genuine and spread the width of his face.

We arrived at the clinic for surgery and my stomach was in knots. I was shuffled off for paperwork and tests.

*   *   *

After I left, my mother cornered Tim.

"You'd better be telling me everything, Timothy," she warned.

"You know everything I know, Elizabeth," he assured her.

"Take out your Bible."

"What?"

"Take out your Bible," she demanded.

Tim's Bible goes everywhere he does. He carries his backpack the way most women carry purses.

He complied.

Mom took it.

"Now put your right hand on it," she instructed.

He did.

"Now, do you solemnly swear that you are telling me the whole story, nothing held back?"

"Elizabeth, why would I....?"

"Swear then!"

"I swear."

"OK," she let the breath she was holding slowly seep out.

"I feel better, now."

Tim's cell phone rang.

"Hello Andrea," he said.

It was my best friend Andrea Cole. And this was about the 17th call of the morning.

"What?" Tim asked.

"You're at St. Luke's?"

"Well, no wonder you can't find us. The surgery is at Mayo."

Andrea is my sister. Well she might as well be. We were college roommates at F.S.U. I know her heart and she knows mine. We are opposites in many ways, even physically. She is very tall, and exotic with long dark hair. She looks like Cher. Andrea is affectionate and caring to the point of obsession. She comes from a big Greek family. I HAVE to tell her everything. She could make coffee nervous.

"It's OK, Andrea," Tim counseled.

"She's fine, just doing pre-op stuff."

Tim knew full well he would be hearing from Andrea another half a dozen times before she got to the clinic. But he had to smile.

"She loves you," he often remarked.

My friend Julie Gillespie was also in the waiting room. Julie and I have known each other since the fifth grade at San Jose Catholic. We went all the way through Bishop Kenny High School together. So much plaid.

Julie is Andrea's polar opposite. My palace guard. She is fiercely protective and no nonsense. Extremely organized. She powers through things the same way I do. We actually became close during my first bout with cancer. She took over my life when I couldn't, and never left my side.

I looked at Julie when I was brought back into the room I called "the holding cell." She looked more nervous than I did.

11

"Smile," I said.

"Oh, I'm fine, I'm fine. You know what my mom always said. 'It's all a giggle.'" She threw her hands in the air. Julie's mom was British. She too suffered from breast cancer, but died from an unrelated illness. Julie was born in England and came to the U.S. as a child.

Last minute hugs all around, and I sat alone with Tim, waiting.

My fingers traced the spot where they would cut. One incision would be made on the right to remove the cancer. Another almost identical one would be needed on the left to insert a port-o-cath. A port was needed for the chemo. I wouldn't be receiving that for a few weeks, but the veins in my arms couldn't take the stress. The port would enter a vein near my heart. A needle would be inserted into the port, accessing the vein during chemo. It leaves a little bulge under the skin that I jokingly called my third boob.

"I'm sorry we have to start our married life this way," I said, tears right on the surface.

Tim put his forehead to mine and laced our fingers together. "We'll be fine darlin'," he said softly.

The door opened and there was Dr. Fulmer, wearing his scrubs and smiling that smile. "I'm sorry," I chimed, "this isn't really a good time for me. Think we could reschedule?"

"Need anything?" he asked.

"A new body and a running cab," I said dryly.

The truth was I was ready to be knocked out. I didn't want to think anymore. I just wanted it to be done. There was no way out of it. So giddyup.

*   *   *

In the waiting room, Andrea was pacing like a rat in a cage. She was devastated that she didn't arrive in time to see me before the surgery, and it was taking much longer than expected.

"I thought this was supposed to be over by now," she groaned. "Where is she?"

12

Tim and Mom were getting anxious too.

"She'll be out soon Andrea," Tim said, as much to convince himself.

Mom was in a trance with her beads, when Dr. Fulmer walked in.

"It went well," he smiled. "It was more complicated than we first imagined, and very tedious trying to get it all, but she did great."

"So…?" My mom wanted to hear that I would live to be a hundred.

"You need to make sure she's aggressive with the follow up treatments," he said. "The chemo and radiation are a must. She's tough, she'll be fine."

"How about long term?" Mom asked.

"She has as much chance of living a long life as any of us," Dr. Fulmer said.

It took me forever to wake up. I kept coming to and fading out. When the world finally came back into focus the news was good and bad. Dr. Fulmer had removed the cancer, but the tiniest tip of the tumor had been touching that vein. Dr. Fulmer pointed to my name on a piece of paper. "See the very top of that "O" in Donna, that's about how much was touching. I scraped it off, but I didn't want to invade the vein itself. We'll have to test it to see if what we scraped had cancer cells. I got all the cancer that I could see."

I tried to swallow the stone in my throat. Another test. Great.

"You wear glasses?" I joked.

True to my word I was back at work the day after my surgery.

I was exhausted, but grateful for the chance to focus on something else. "Hey Donna, how ya' doin'?"

"Good to see you back." Shouts of welcome were coming from the newsroom. "Geez Hicken, you slacker, couldn't you come back sooner?"

Kim Romano turned her head from her computer at the assignment desk. "I sent you a few e-mails," she said.

I rounded the turn to my desk and my heart flipped.

"It looks like a shrine," I thought.

13

Flowers, cookies, teddy bears, balloons, notes. All from viewers. I surveyed the desk for a few moments, shaking my head.

"People are incredible," I said aloud.

After looking over my new treasure, I sat down to log on to my computer.

"Lord have mercy," I mouthed.

E-mails. Hundreds of them sat waiting to put their arms around me.

To: donnahicken@firstcoastnews.com
Subject: Thought, prayers... and admiration

Donna,

I know you are surely receiving hundreds and hundreds of e-mails, and I can't recall that I have ever once taken time to convey personal wishes to anyone I do not personally know, but I feel compelled to join others in wishing you very quick and lasting health. Your strength and determination have been such an inspiration to me and my friends, yet I know there must be many frightening and dark moments.

I am about your age with an often all-too-consuming job, and I'm a single mother. (We were pregnant at the same time, and I recall being mildly irritated by how great you looked the whole time....)

I do well to cope with the routine everyday challenges, but about a month ago, I went through the whole mammogram-to-biopsy nightmare. Only by grace though, I was a lucky one. ....benign. I often thought about you that entire week-and-a-half of being near breathless with fear. I steeled myself and was fully prepared to fight and win, if forced to. (...and wondered if my hair could ever look as great as yours did at an inch-long).

I wish you the continued resolve and strength to fight like hell, and will hope and pray that life may quickly return to whatever feels like "normal" for you and your family.
Sincere and warm wishes.
Sonya Doerr
Ponte Vedra Beach

To: donnahicken@firstcoastnews.com
Subject: Prayers

Dear Donna,
I just had to write and tell you that you are in my thoughts and prayers. I saw your beautiful segment the other night sharing your most recent news. You are so brave. I am going through breast cancer right now. I am the third daughter out of five to be diagnosed in the past ten years. We are all under forty so they are trying to figure out what's going on! We are all doing well so far.

You seem like such a beautiful, gracious person. I just want you to know how many of us are pulling for you. You are our role model! I wish you the very best.

Hopefully, some of my hair will grow back in time for my son's graduation from Bolles (sorry, I know you went to B.K.) on the 25th. I have had tremendous support from the people in the Bolles family - especially the baseball family (my son Jon pitches for Bolles). I also have a twelve year old daughter. The kids are doing very well with it so far. Please let me know if I can ever do anything for you. God bless you.
Sincerely,
Wendi Hollis

To: donnahicken@firstcoastnews.com
Subject: MY PRAYERS

Donna,
My prayers are with you. May God bless and keep you. I am sure that you will beat this after all you already have.

I am a survivor of 7 years. First, I lost a finger to melanoma in January of 1995. I also had to have a limpafusion in April of that year. In 1997 they found a tumor in my lower back that was inoperable, I had radiation and 15 bottles of Interleukin-2. In 1999 I had breast cancer another 34 days of radiation. I am 57 years old and I refuse to have it again. I have 2 children and 5 grandchildren and I live each and every day for them.

If you ever need a friend to just talk to or pray with I would be happy to do this for you. I watch you on the news and I admire you so much. Just hang in there because you WILL WIN. Always remember that God only gives us what He thinks that we can handle sometimes I feel like He thinks that I have the shoulders of a line backer but only He knows for sure. I also think that you are a beautiful and very graceful lady. And I liked you with no hair.
Again may God bless and keep you and your family always.
Nancy Wood (Macclenny, FL)

To: news@firstcoastnews.com
Subject: Donna Hicken

Was wondering if Donna Hicken's story and progress will be posted on your website?
Thanks
Lois Stanford

"Tim, people are so good to me. You've got to read some of this stuff," I said at dinner. "You're not going to believe it."

The truth is, Tim has never had a difficult time believing good things about people. He's a meteorologist. I'm a journalist.

"Of course I believe it," he said. "Are you going to say something on the air?"

"Briefly," I said. "But I don't want to talk about it on the air too much. It makes the news about me, and not about the news. Know what I mean?"

"Yeah…," he nodded, then paused. Tim always does this when he's going to argue the point.

"You'll find a good balance. People want to know how you are."

"So do I," I thought.

"One viewer wondered if I might post my progress on the web. I'm thinking maybe a weekly journal, we'll see."

The tests showed there were cancer cells present where the tumor touched the vein, but Dr. Fulmer felt that the cells had not gone through the vein itself.

"So," said Edith, my chart spread in front of her. "Instead of starting with the chemo this time, we are going to start with radiation."

The idea was to destroy the remaining cells on the surface without causing too much damage to the vein. Not easy.

In my mind I could see them marching, these nasty invaders, toward the open highway of my body.

"Can we start now?" I asked.

"I want you to meet with Dr. Collie," said Edith. "He'll be your radiation oncologist."

Dr. Collie reminds me of a hard-driving southern football coach. I was the star player and he was Bear Bryant.

"OK Donna, we've got our team together," he announced. "Here's the game plan." He proceeded to show me all my CT images. I would have to have more to map out my body intricately so that the radiation could be directed to the exact spot where the cells still existed. "And we're just gonna blast away at it!" When he finished in the huddle and left the room, I looked at Tim and we both started to laugh. "OK, ready?" he chanted. "One, two, three. Break!"

That would be our chant every time a meeting with Dr. Collie was discussed.

TWO

I'm Radioactive

"I will make myself healthy.
I will make myself stronger.
I will beat this disease.
I am strong.
I am determined."

Morning convictions. This was the assignment from my personal trainer Brett Chepenik.

"You have got to take the word "can't" out of your vocabulary, Donna," Brett instructed as we began our morning workout. "It's self-defeating."

Brett is a big believer in positive thinking. He helps me fight gravity, both inside and out.

Tall and muscular, with his shaved head Brett might look intimidating if you couldn't see his face. It shines with assurance and optimism. I'm not sure the man is capable of a negative thought.

I settled under the bench press.

"OK, here we go," he urged.

The right side of my chest struggled to come along with the left. The surgery left me much weaker there.

"Just ten, just get ten," Brett prompted, and started to count down to one.

"Three, two, who's your favorite?" He taunted.

I always think if I could just put Brett in my pocket to be pulled out every time I have a confidence crisis, life would be much easier.

19

The next morning would be one of those times.

The start of radiation. My coach was waiting.

The hallway to the radiation area is endless. Radiology is at the far north end of the Mayo Clinic. Walking to it this first day was a flashback.

"Wasn't I just here?" I said to Tim.

We turned left into the waiting room.

"Good morning, do you have your schedule?" The same pleasant woman from two years ago was at the desk. As she checked me in, I could hear my name echoed in whispers behind me.

I grabbed a magazine. "Foods that fight cancer," blared the headline on the front. I put it back down. I looked up to see a nice 60-something woman walking toward me. She reached out and took my hand.

"Dear, I hope you don't mind my interruption," she said. "I just want you to know that I'm praying for you."

"Thank you so much," I replied. "I'll take all of those I can get. And how are you doing?"

"Oh, I'm just waiting for my husband. He's doing fine."

So often, this was the kind of answer I got from people. They didn't seem to want to burden me with their own troubles. I wished they would. I don't want people to have the notion that, because I'm on TV, I think my worries are somehow more significant than theirs.

"Donna Hicken," the voice was coming from a nurse at the door to the treatment rooms.

"Sounds like me," I said. "Thank you so much for the prayers."

We were escorted to Dr. Collie's office.

"OK, Donna, I think we've got a winner here," he said.

"I've been going over the plan with the whole team. We think the most effective way to do this is to attack the cancer from two fronts. The radiation can actually be enhanced by the kind of chemo you're going to have. So we are going to do them both at once."

"At the same time?" I asked, about an octave higher than normal.

20

I had psyched myself up for radiation. It's really a walk in the park next to chemo. Makes me a little tired, and it's a grind to have it every single day, scary to think of it in my body, but besides giving me a "sunburn," it's not unbearable.

Chemo, on the other hand, is pure hell. Worse. Someone sneaks into my body, possesses it, sucks the life out of it and leaves me to deal with the shell. It leeches the hope right out of my soul.

"I thought I had six weeks before I'd start chemo," I said.

"Dr. Perez will explain more," he said. "But this will get us to our goal faster."

"Wish I could punt," I thought.

Dr. Collie led me back to a room where they would take "one more picture" of my chest to make sure the radiation would be delivered to the right place.

"You'll have to stay out here," the nurse said to Tim.

My chest tightened. Tim was with me for everything. I suddenly felt insecure.

"Why?" I asked.

"We don't want him exposed to the radiation," she said.

Having already been through six weeks of radiation the first time, now facing six more, this was not a comforting statement.

"Hey," I said, "my radiation is his radiation."

The nurse smiled blandly and turned to Tim. "I'll have her out in a few minutes."

Inside the room I was the human drawing board. The tech drew what amounts to a map on my chest with a black permanent marker. An X over the spot where we'd be "blasting away."

"OK, Miss Donna, we're set. Ready for your tattoo?"

"Sure," I said. "How about a little butterfly on my left shoulder? I've always thought that might be nice."

God bless these ladies. Don't you know how many times they have probably heard lame jokes like that from nervous cancer patients. But they were kind enough to laugh.

With radiation, tattoos serve as crosshairs of sorts. It's how they line up the beams to make sure they zap you in the intended

21

places. The tattoos are no larger than the period on the end of this sentence. They are with you forever. The mark of the beast.

Back into my favorite backless gown and terry cloth robe, I was helped up onto the table for my first treatment.

"Arms over your head, Donna, try to relax," the tech said.

I placed my arms in my very own plastic mold and tried to breath. Each patient has to have a custom mold made. It means your position never changes from week to week. This is a business of millimeters.

"Some people like to save these for souvenirs when their treatment is over," she said.

How sentimental.

She stepped outside and talked with me through a microphone from a "safe room." Once again, I was left alone with my radiation.

The large machine started to click and buzz over me.

"Relax, just relax, breath normally," I told myself. The tech told me not to worry about holding my breath because it wouldn't matter.

"Why not?" I thought. "If I have to have tattoos, and we're worried about millimeters, why won't my breathing throw things off?"

I held my breath whenever possible. I could count the cycles. The first blast was short, just a few seconds. The machine rotated. The second one longer, about 45. Click. The third longer still. Eight in all.

"Don't hyperventilate," I thought. "Don't move."

Finally, it was over. It could have been days. It was only three minutes.

"That's it, girl, one down. See you tomorrow," she said.

"And the next day, and the next day and the next," I thought. I would have to have 33 treatments in all.

"How are you?" Tim asked, as I walked out.

"I'm radioactive," I said. I broke into that 80s song by The Firm.

"I'm not uptight, not unattractive, turn me on tonight, I'm

22

radioactive, radioactive...."

"Who was the guitar player?" Tim loves to quiz me on music.

"I don't.... wait a minute, Jimmy Page."

"Veeery good," he said.

Walking back down the long hallway I counted my steps.

"Don't look at the end, Donna, just one foot in front of the other," I told myself. "Think of this as your marathon. You're at the starting line. You are just beginning. You aren't even thinking about the finish. It's a long way. Just go."

Tim and I had planned to run the Chicago Marathon in October. Now that would have to wait.

I love running marathons. Twenty-six-point-two miles of pure will. I relish the challenge of it. The sweat. Making it through the pain. Feeling there's nothing left and then pushing through to the other side. The pure joy and satisfaction of the finish. I start slow as mud, people streaming past me. But step by step I pass a lot of them during the race. They come out too fast, get caught up in trying to outpace the guy next to them. I outlast them. I endure. I'm never going to be competition for anybody, just myself, and that's enough.

"You can do this," I thought.

We got to the elevators and took one to the eighth floor to meet with Edith. She was relieved that we didn't have to wait for the end of radiation to begin the chemotherapy.

"This is good, Donna, very good. I didn't want to wait," she said.

"We'll give your body another week to recover from the surgery then we'll begin."

I had to ask the question. It had been burning in my brain from the time Edith told me the cancer didn't recur, but was there all along.

"What makes you think it will work this time? If those other cells were left, obviously it didn't..."

"It didn't work," Edith completed my sentence.

"Well, for one thing, as you know, we are not using the same drugs. You will receive paclitaxel and carboplatin. They are excellent drugs and they break down cancer cells in a totally different way, than the drugs you had before.

"But there's no guarantee they will work," I said.

"That is the tough thing about cancer, Donna, these treatments don't always work. But they are the best tools we have."

*   *   *

Why is it those things we dread always come faster than those we desire?

The first day of chemo arrived in a split-second.

My phone rang at 6:30 a.m. It was Tim.

"Can I read you something?" he asked.

I smiled. This had become a bit of a morning ritual.

"Faith does not do away with our human condition, our limited vision, our wavering mind, but it does give us the power to walk where the earth is not firm, to see where the air is not clear, to set sail when the sea is not calm; the power to hope in the midst of despondency, to love in the midst of indifference, to smile in the midst of misunderstanding. We remain very much in the world, but we have a glimpse of the truth that is clear and firm and eternal, and with that gentle ray of light we direct our steps through the surrounding darkness. Faith is not an insurance policy but a courageous adventure, not a tranquilizer but a challenge, not a bed of roses but a battlefront. Faith does not take away the veil of mystery but teaches us to look through it in wonder and hope. The true understanding of faith prepares the mind for the risks of life under God's loving gaze."

The passage was written by a priest, Father Carlos Valles. It's entitled "Let go of Fear." Tim and I read it one day, months before, in a book of daily scripture readings called *Living Faith*. It had become our mantra for all kinds of reasons.

On the drive into Mayo we said almost nothing.

24

"Mile one, Donna," I thought. "Just get this one out of the way."

"Hi there Kids!" I beamed as we entered the chemo floor.

"Miss me?" I looked around at the warm, friendly faces of my angels. Many of the chemo nurses who had cared for me the first time were still there. There was Rini and Lori, Beth, and of course, there was Aurora. I call her the Spanish whirlwind.

Aurora is not a nurse. She's a volunteer supreme. She was diagnosed with a vicious cancer called multiple myeloma, six years before I met her. They gave her six months. She withstood more than a year of grueling treatments that would kill most people's will to live. She is the first to tell you that she "kicked cancer's butt."

"I'ma nah supposa have a beer when I'ma treated," she loved to recount in her broken English. "Mah huzbun woulda tell on me to mah Doctor. But mah Doctor woulda say, whatevera maka her feela better. So ah say whata da hell, one beer maka me feel good, three maka me feel better." Aurora has the most infectious laugh. I call her Aurora Borealis. She is a light in the gloom for sure. It is impossible to have an ounce of self-pity when she's around.

"Gimme a hug, girl," she demanded, stretching out her arms to me.

"We are tough you and me. It'sah gonna be fine."

I settled into room number three and waited like a death row inmate for the warden to call it all off.

The room was cold. Anything below 80º is cold to me.

"Want me to find you a blanket?" Tim asked.

"That would help, thanks."

When Tim returned the nurse followed him into the room.

"Goooood morning. Are we ready to party?"

His name was Jim. A burly man with salt and pepper hair, who gave the impression he was right where he wanted to be.

"She's ready," Tim answered for me.

He took the seat across from mine and smiled back at me.

"Why not," I said.

"So do you want the freezy spray?" Jim asked.

25

The "freezy spray" is a numbing agent, which when applied to the port, makes the needle prick less painful. The port needle is fairly large and has a slight bend at the end.

"Of course I want it," I said. "When I was pregnant I asked the doctor to start the epidural at my 37 week check up. I'm a wimp."

"I'm with you," Jim said.

He sprayed my skin with the cold liquid.

"Ready, deep breath." He pushed the needle through. "And we're in."

"My God," I thought. "I'm really doing this again."

A shiver ran through my body as the first cool fluids flowed into my veins.

First the saline for hydration. Then the Tagamet so the drugs wouldn't give me indigestion. Then Zofran, so I wouldn't throw up. Then steroids, also for nausea and to stave off any allergic reaction. Then Benadryl, another medication to block my body's insistence that this poison doesn't belong.

After all the pre-meds were "on board" Jim talked about cancer. About how sorry he was that I had to go through this again, and how a positive attitude is important. Then, for no apparent reason, I started giggling. Then laughing. Then full-on-tears-in-the-eyes-howling. I couldn't help it. It was like someone was tickling me.

Tim looked at me, stunned. My laughter couldn't have been more inappropriate. Here was Jim, discussing a perfectly serious topic, and I was gonzo.

Tim let out an uncomfortable laugh and looked at Jim.

"It's the Benadryl," Jim said chuckling. "I'll try to give it slower next time, but that happens to a lot of people."

It wore off after a minute or two, but it happened at every chemo treatment from May through October.

"Time for the yucky stuff," Jim said.

I took a deep breath. Slowly, the alien began its possession. My enemy and my friend. The paclitaxel, more commonly known as Taxol, has to invade slowly. It took nearly an hour to flow in. Then the carboplatin. A small bag that packed a nauseating punch.

26

One drug would disable the monster, the other would cut its head off.

The entire treatment took three hours.

"I need to stop and get my Zofran prescription filled," I told Tim on the way home. "And my steroids."

I would have to take three Zofran tablets a day for three days after chemo to keep my stomach in check. Steroids were stepped down over two days for the same purpose.

I went into the pharmacy while Tim waited in the car. Moments later I returned with my stash.

"Well," I said. "Thank goodness we have this prescription card to pay for the drugs."

"How much?" Tim asked.

"Oh, I only paid $15. Without the card, are you ready for this? It would have been $2,200."

"Are you serious?"

"Perfectly. What in the world do people do when they don't have insurance?"

"Man," Tim shook his head. "No kidding."

I went home and slept for the rest of the day until it was time to go to work. I was just starting to feel that cloud passing over my body. The first day after chemo and into the second, it's not that bad. Just a dull sense of nausea and an overall malaise. It's the third day, when the steroids are gone that the drugs really take hold. It's a 90 mile per hour ride into a brick wall. Fatigue so total it defies description. A tidal wave of nausea. A hollowness both physical and emotional that simply cannot be filled.

I sat down to check the rundown for the 5:30 show, and made a few changes to my scripts.

"How many times have I got to say "a lot" is two words, not "alot," I said to no one.

I finished with the copy and popped anxiously into my e-mail. This was now the highlight of my days. I always was tempted to go there first. It was such a lift. I was working feverishly to answer as many as I could, but I was falling behind. The ones I wanted to answer most were the ones where people asked me not to burden myself with responding. It was no burden. These faceless friends were becoming my lifeline.

To: donnahicken@firstcoastnews.com
Subject: Thank You

Dear Donna,
My name is Dan Stovall and last year I called you because my wife (Carol) had been diagnosed with breast cancer and needed someone to talk to. You were kind enough to call back and talk to her on the phone. I know I am way late in telling you this, but that call REALLY helped her a lot. She had so many questions about what was going to happen and you were able to help her understand what was going to happen and what to expect. It's been a tough eighteen months but she is still here and taking it one day at a time. We, of course, have been keeping up with you and your fight with cancer. So I just wanted you to know that you are always in our prayers and I know you probably don't need it but we are here for you if you need us. I will forever be in your debt for what you did for Carol and if there is ever anything I can do for you PLEASE let me know.
Thanks again for everything.
Dan Stovall

To: Dan Stovall
Subject: RE: Thank You

Hi Dan,
Thanks so much for the kind words. I'm glad that in some way I can help. Your thoughts and prayers will be plenty

for me... believe me. I pray you and your family are well. Tell your wife to keep the faith...I'm still here if she needs me!
Donna

To: donnahicken@firstcoastnews.com
Subject: Thoughts & Prayers

Dear Donna:
I know you probably do get hundreds (or maybe even thousands) of e-mails from your fans and folks that want you to know they are in your corner, but I just could not resist.

When I first moved back to Jacksonville in 1999, I didn't know any of the newscasters (imagine that, I'd only been gone 15 years), but as time moved on, I learned more and more about the different personalities. One of things that impressed me most about you was that despite your trials and tribulations, you continued to "push." I admire that and cannot even imagine being able to conduct myself in the same manner.

You are a very special person in many, many ways. Every time I'm handed something that I don't think I can handle, I think about you and what you've been able to handle and smack myself in the face and go forward.

My prayers and thoughts are with you... keep pushin' girl, you've got a lot to do in this world.
Anjie Chapman

To: Anjie Chapman
Subject: Thank you

Anjie,
Thank goodness I haven't done my make-up yet. You'd
have made my mascara run. Your letter was so kind and
I can't tell you how much it means to me that you would
take the time to write. I'm sure if you were in my shoes
you'd do just the same thing. After all what choice do we
have when faced with adversity but to face it right back.
I've got two little kids who wouldn't let me think about
anything else! Thanks so much for the nice thoughts.
God bless.
Donna

Out of the several dozen new e-mails from the day before, I
was able to answer five or six before it was time to get ready for
the broadcast.

I could hear Tim in my ear whenever I failed to write someone
back.

"They'll want to know how you're doing."

Maybe I should follow through on that journal idea...

After the show, I turned to the one person who I knew could
help get me started. Then I sat down to tap out an e-mail to my
boss.

To: McCormick, Mike
Subject: web journal

Mike... I've had so many requests from people for health
updates and I don't want to get into doing anything on
the air.... but... I had a long talk with my friend Wendy

Chioji in Orlando tonight and she has a journal on the station's web site.... She writes in it once a week about her breast cancer experience.... and viewers can communicate with her that way and they feel updated. I would be willing to do something like that if you thought it was appropriate. I can't keep up with all the e-mail. I'm trying to answer it all... But this might be easier... what do you think? I will talk with Thomas if you give me the go ahead.

Mike loved the idea.

My friend Wendy Chioji is an anchor for WESH in Orlando. She wrote an on-line journal during her own battle with breast cancer to deal with the same issues. I dialed the extension for Thomas Wilson our webmaster.

"Hi Thomas, it's Donna. I'm calling to make more work for you," I said.

"I'm always looking for more work," he answered. "What's up?"

I explained the journal and asked him to check out the WESH site to get some ideas. I would write in it once a week to update folks on my progress and people could e-mail me through the journal site.

"Sounds cool," he said. "I'll get it set up and you can see what you think."

For the next few days the journal was not at the top of my priority list.

It was a short list. Get out of bed. Don't throw up. Impersonate a human being to Tim and the kids. Do the news. Make it to the end of the broadcast at 11:35 p.m. Say goodnight.

Soon I had to add another item. Take a dust buster to my pillow case.

The following week, after my second chemo treatment, it started. Just a few strands at first. Then clumps. The station wanted

31

me to hold off on shaving my head for as long as possible. I hadn't been able to find a wig I liked. I was hoping to keep my hair this time. With Taxol, some women do. Not me. By the end of the second week, I couldn't take it anymore. My scalp was visible from all angles. I had searched and searched for a wig and finally settled on a head of long blonde hair. My real hair was about an inch long all over my head. The "powers that be" weren't thrilled, but they were trying to be sensitive. I was emotionally overwrought. Absolutely beside myself when I sat down in the general manager's office.

Ken Tonning has always been good to me, as has Gannett, the company that owns the station. I'm not a person who goes into Ken's office much. If I do, it's usually something serious.

"Ken, I can't do this anymore," I sobbed. Poor Ken. I was practically hysterical.

"Of course, I wouldn't ask you to do that, Donna," he said, trying his best to comfort me. "We'll go with the wig today."

I cried all the way to the Casa Blanca Salon and my stylist, Lisa shaved the remaining stragglers. She helped me fit the wig to my head and "Brenda" was born.

"You have to say her name in a breathy way," I joked with co-anchor, Phil Amato, pulling myself back together before the show. "She's Brhhhendah."

I was starting to feel better. It was a relief to get rid of that sign of my sickness. Brenda represented a lively, more youthful me, until the old Donna could return.

My colleague, Jeannie Blaylock and I did the honors of introducing Brenda to the viewers. We did a mini-interview on chairs next to the set.

The camera started on her. "As you know, Donna is going through treatment for breast cancer," she said into the camera. "And she's decided to go with a different look while she's waiting for her hair to grow back."

The camera panned wide to show me sitting there wearing Brenda.

"If you don't like it, don't call me," I said. "You'll hurt my feelings." I smiled, but the truth is I meant it. I was insecure enough.

The phones started ringing off the hook. And the e-mails. Oh my gosh, the e-mails. It seemed everyone had an opinion.

To: donnahicken@firstcoastnews.com
Subject: 'from Donna's Journal'

Donna,
You look MAAAAAAAAARVELOUS!!!! May God bless you and your family!
Take care,
Dayzie Nieves (Lawtey, FL)

To: donnahicken@firstcoastnews.com
Subject: 'from Donna's Journal'

Dear Donna:

I hope this finds you well and your spirits are up. And by the way, you are still the prettiest woman on the News! I don't know if you ever saw the film clip of me when the Robert Myer Hotel was demolished, but I was the cop who replied to the camera, "Donna Hicken is a major babe." "Brenda" looks good on you. My sister went through chemo and had her wigs as well. It seemed that each wig gave her a different personality, confirming what I had always teased her about being Schizophrenic. She had a very aggressive type and fought a good fight. Her beauty and personality really shown through during those times and I was very fortunate to be her brother.

If there was something I could say to you personally, I guess it would be, even though you see so many wonderful

33

gestures of affection and friendship coming from everyone, you are only seeing maybe 20% of what is actually there. My sister knew how I felt, but there was so much more inside me that she didn't see. When I graduated from the Police Academy and received my badge, I wanted her to be the first one to pin it on me. Seeing her come into the auditorium on her crutches and sitting in the front row overshadowed everything else that day. I was so proud of her, she was a much braver person that I will ever be.

I just wanted you to know that everyone is pulling for you and that if you ever get down, and feel weakened, many of us are getting strength through your courage and bright spirit. We are with you all the way. It is a pleasure watching you work on the newscast. I see my sister in you everyday.

If there is anything I can ever do for you, as a person or a Police Officer, just let me know and it's done. Even if you do wear Garnet & Gold, I still think you are a major babe.
Best wishes,
Ed

To: Ed
Subject: re: 'from Donna's Journal'

Ed....
what a beautiful letter. I'm sure your sister still sees and feels how much you love her. I'm honored you see her in me. Thank you so much for taking the time to write and for recalling things that must still be difficult. As for the "major babe" part... I don't think I've ever felt less attractive in my life... but hey... if you like bald girls... I won't complain!

34

Keep taking care of our great city and again... thank you for your kind words.
Donna

To: donnahicken@firstcoastnews.com
Subject: Donna, AKA, Brenda

We, and God, are with you, but we HATE the long wig. Please find a short one, or let us see you without any hair. You are beautiful with short hair, and will be with NO hair. The wig makes you look weird.
Thanks,
and may God bless.
Libby and Leonard Wells

To: LIBBY&LEONARD
Subject: RE: Donna, AKA, Brenda

Hi Libby and Leonard!
Thanks for taking the time to write. I'm sorry you hate the wig.
I tried to find a short one... But none was anywhere near like my real hair and those I tried really looked awful. If I could go on bald I would... but that would make the news more about my bald head than what it should be about. I can't really win with the hair at this point.
Truthfully with all that's going on in my life right now... it's not too high on my priority list. I'm afraid we'll all have to live with it for a while. Weird or not... I hope you'll still tune in.
Donna

To: donnahicken@firstcoastnews.com
Subject: Your Wig Looks Great

Dear Donna, I think your wig looks just great. When ya'll were showing flashbacks for the 10th anniversary of Buddy Check 12 you and Jeanie looked great. When I saw you with the wig on it reminded me of you a few years ago. I pray for you every day. You look really great !!!!!!!!!!! I have been a fan of yours since you came on the news, God Bless!!!!!!!!!
Hayley Young

To: <news@firstcoastnews.com>
Subject: Hair

Donna - Way to go Champ - I admire your courage and spunk. Prayers and love are with you during these trying times. Your hair looks great but your attitude is greater.
Pat Moitt

To: donnahicken@firstcoastnews.com
Subject: hooray!

Dear Donna,
I just wanted you to know that you are truly one of the most courageous women I have "known." You are an inspiration to so many!! As a Jacksonville native, I have watched you from the beginning. I love watching you in the evening and on the late broadcast as well. I just wanted to wish you well and let you know that our prayers are with you. I cried when you made the announcement

that your cancer had come back, and then cheered
knowing that you truly will beat this!!! I love the new hair
by the way :-) Take care and God Bless!!
Kimberly Osborne

There was even one from across the river. My friend and
competitor, Channel 4 anchor Deborah Gianoulis, sent this note
of encouragement:

To: donnahicken@firstcoastnews.com
Subject: Donna's Hair

Dear Donna, You look like a teenager again. You could
put on that Bishop Kenny uniform and take classes!
God Bless you!
Deborah G.

To: DeborahGianoulis
Subject: RE: Donna's Hair

Deb you are so kind. I cried all day. Didn't want to lose
the last few strands of my hair... didn't want to wear the
wig. No choice in either! Anyhow it's a fun wig as wigs
go. Thanks for the encouragement... hope all is well with
you and your family.
Donna

To: donnahicken@firstcoastnews.com
Subject: Donna's Hair

Dear Donna,
Honest to God, the wig is cute. I can't imagine how sick of this you must be. I have read that book "Why Bad Things Happen to Good People" and I still can't say that I understand. Do you have any insights after all you have been through? My kids are well. How about yours? I know they must keep you going.
Love, Deb

To: DeborahGianoulis
Subject: RE: Donna's Hair

Hi Deb...
You said it. The kids are all I can think about through all of this. It's tough for me to do this in such a fishbowl... but even tougher for them. They've been little troopers though. Danielle hates the long hair... Drew loves it. That's a man for you! They seem to be taking it mostly in stride though. I think watching me come through it OK before has helped. I don't know what to say about insights except that I have never really asked God why. I figure bad things happen to all of us. I just look to God for the strength to face it with some grace. The weekend I was first diagnosed... Tim took me to mass at the basilica and the whole homily was about embracing our crosses instead of just carrying them. I felt like the priest was talking right to me. So to that end... I am starting a foundation for women who can't afford breast cancer treatment. You wouldn't believe the horror stories out there. It's also a way for me to find some positive out of all this. Oh so sorry to ramble. You wind me up and I just don't stop! All

in all life's good kiddo. The docs tell me this is just a local thing and they are hoping this does the trick. Me too!!!! Take care... and I'd love your input on the foundation if you have any thoughts. I'm in the process of incorporating right now... but could sure use some advice. Take care.
Love,
Donna

The following week, Donna's Journal was born.

Donna's Journal
Home>Health Watch
June 10, 2002

Hi folks!

I have gotten so many e-mails and words of encouragement from you... and I can't begin to thank you enough. You have no idea how much strength all the prayers and thoughts give me. I am trying to answer when I can... sometimes I get a little overwhelmed so please try to be patient with me. I am going to use this site as a journal of sorts because many of you have asked what's happening with me.

First of all... thanks for caring so much. You often mention that I seem like family... and you are like that to me too. I have just finished my first full round of chemo treatments... I have either three or five left depending on what the doc decides.

The wig... like it or not... will be with us for a while. The great majority of you have had kind words for her. I call her "Brenda." If you liked the short hair better... well just indulge me for a while. It makes me feel good.

My cancer was localized and removed... and my doc says my prognosis is good. Obviously I would have preferred not to travel this path again... but God has plans for me.

I am working on some exciting stuff that I hope will help a lot of other women going through this... but more on that later. I'll be writing in this journal every week so stay tuned... and again... thank you so much for taking the time to let me know you care. It means so much.

Your biggest fan,

Donna

THREE

The Loaves and the Fishes

The journal entries started as a means of convenient communication. What they became was a certifiable "loaves and fishes" miracle. I sent out this tiny basket, with a small sincere offering inside. I received, in return, a feast beyond what I could possibly consume.

To: donnahicken@firstcoastnews.com
Subject: Thinking of you

Dear Donna,
You interviewed me prior to the RITA race of 2001. My name is Laura Heyler and at the time I was just finishing up my treatment for breast cancer. Our paths crossed momentarily after that interview at a Jags game and at another fund raising event. I want you to know how important you have become to me. After meeting you for the first time I was moved by your spirit, you have an inner source of magnetism that touches others. The sincerity and grounding of your personality is both comforting and motivating.

After the on air announcement of your recurrence I cried with you, for you, and for those whom you have touched. I have no doubt that you will be a survivor again. Viewing the changes in you while you undergo therapy is difficult.

41

From a personal standpoint, I am terrified of a recurrence in myself. It is also difficult to think of you on a daily basis and wondering how you are feeling and knowing that you must function in your busy life while fighting cancer again.

I pray for you and know that you will again be healed. Thank you for being so strong and beautiful.
With Feeling-
Laura Heyler

To: donnahicken@firstcoastnews.com
Subject: Hope you are feeling OK!

Donna,
I was taken away when I heard that you were battling Cancer again. I can only imagine how hard that must be. You are a wonderful person I am sure, just from watching how caring you are on the news. I just want to send along my best wishes for you. I know lots of prayers are being sent out for you! God has you in his arms at this trying time. Keep your head up. My thoughts and prayers are also with you. Best Wishes.
Sarah Anderson (St. Augustine FL,)

To: donnahicken@firstcoastnews.com
Subject: 'from Donna's Journal'

Good luck and God bless you as you continue to fight your cancer. You are an inspiration to many and you seem to have avoided becoming a "victim" to this process. Hang in there! We all eagerly await the next hairdo! I am a nurse practitioner in a family practice office. I have many patients in various stages of dealing with breast cancer. I recently came upon a problem that amazes me, and that you might be able to influence. One of my patients had a mastectomy last year, with the removal of lymph nodes. She now has a condition called lymphedema, which causes her affected arm to swell because the lymph fluid cannot get out easily through these surgically affected lymph channels. There is therapy for it, and special dressings to wear that reduce the swelling and promote lymph flow. However, insurance doesn't pay for this therapy, the Cancer Society will not subsidize it because it requires the use of supplies (dressings), and it is a long-term condition. I wonder why needy patients can get wigs, bras, etc., but not the needed therapy (10-12 visits) or the dressings. No other funding sources seem to fit here either. I just found out about a Lymphedema group located in Orange Park, and will contact them, but this seems like one of those ever-enlarging "cracks" that many patients/people slip through. Maybe some of your audience has some experience with lymphedema treatments and can help.

Good luck in dealing with your illness! You are a role model!

Pat Richards

"Hi buddy, I'm just calling to check-in on you," Andrea's voice on my phone message service. "Try to call me back, please, I've been trying to reach you for days."

Beep.

"Hey, it's me." Julie's voice next. "Have you fallen off the face of the earth or what? Call me."

I can't explain the loneliness. These women are my closest girl friends and yet I couldn't talk to them. I told myself it was because no one could understand. But that wasn't it.

I couldn't even talk to my Boston buddy Nancy Bauer. She and I were battling at the same time. We had met when we were both training to run the Boston Marathon in 1999. Ironically we were running for Dana-Farber, a cancer institute in Boston. Then Nancy was already dealing with her first diagnosis of breast cancer. She actually conquered the infamous "Heart Break Hill" during her chemotherapy! Amazing. I would be diagnosed months later, but was surely already carrying the disease around in my body. Nancy came to Jacksonville for the Gate River Run the last week of my first round of chemotherapy in 2000. She had just had surgery for a recurrence. We ran the 9.3 mile course slowly but triumphantly together. How, I still don't know, but we were quite the pair.

If anyone understood my mental state, Nancy did. And my silence hurt. She tried to reach me by phone for weeks, then e-mail. She even called Tim to make sure I was alive. Finally, I e-mailed her back to apologize and ask her not to be angry. This is what I received in return.

To: donnahicken@firstcoastnews.com
Subject: Warm Thoughts

Hi back atcha -
I am sitting here in my office drinking with my Cinnamon Toast coffee in my Shelby's Coffee Shoppe mug. Please forgive me if the perception of the messages I have left have been that I am angry for you not calling. I know you well enough by now and vice versa to realize how we both deal with what we are going through. You are right - to hear our voices together talking can bring a lot of strength to each other whereby we can at least find some sort of humor in all of this. But I am finding it harder and harder to find any humor and am reaching in more and more and not reaching out - believe it or not. This is all kind of new for me.

I hope you are not angry that I called Tim - even hearing

44

his voice tell me you are hanging in and getting through brought comfort. He told me how Drew and Danielle were learning to surf - what a hoot and something that must bring you much joy and laughter. I hope to see that and them next week, it's been so long. You and I both know it's sometimes easier to hear and know that neither of us are alone in these pains of life and in no way do I feel that by not speaking to each other on the phone, that it is meant to be punishment. Hell, we could just sit and drink coffee, not say anything and just nod our freakin blonde heads, and know that each understands the other and maybe laugh at each other too.

Again, please accept my apology for the rudeness of my message yesterday. It was a bad moment and I let out my anger and fear of that moment on you in my message and I am sorry. You know what's going on with me, I know what's going on with you too and we can share our war stories next week.

In any event, I leave Sunday for Jackson, MS where I hear it is a balmy 50 degrees (ya right!) and arrive in Jacksonville late Tuesday night. I really just hope to sit my behind on the beach with a couple of books and relax for as long as I possibly can. If I can get a decent night's sleep that would be a bonus.

Hope you are out on the beach taking a nice walk or just sipping some coffee and being good to yourself - you deserve that Donna and more. Looking forward to having coffee together - nah, let's do wine - next week.

Sending you very warm thoughts and lotsa love - every day !!
Love, Nancy

Nancy was always much better at reaching out than I was. My instinct was to isolate. It wasn't personal. It was survival in my world.

"Can't you tell I'm trying my best to tread water," I thought. "Just leave me alone."

Funny thing was, I could talk to the viewers writing in. With them, I shared my fears, and vented my frustrations. They did the same, sharing with me the most intimate pain of their own struggles. We talked about faith and strength and fighting back and love. And we laughed too. My least personal relationships were my greatest source of comfort. My life boat.

Things around me were sinking.

"Your white count is too low, Donna. I can't treat you this week," Edith said on the phone.

Each week I had bloodwork to make sure my counts were hanging in there. If my white count was below 1.0 chemo was cancelled. Too risky. Nothing left to fight infection. It was a risk even to be at work. I had to ask my co-workers to keep away from my desk.

To: news-all@firstcoastnews.com
Subject: BUBBLE GIRL

Hi kids..... Sicko here.

Listen, I know you all are aware that my desk is the most sterile environment one could imagine... But here's the deal. Because of my chemo, my white blood count... which for all you journalism majors means the cells that fight infection... has gone down to statistical zero. That means if I get sick I go to the hospital. Soooooooooo if you don't mind please don't use my phone or my computer. I'll just keep my germs to myself.

Yours in chemicals,
Donna

The first time I was diagnosed, my counts did the same thing. Statistical Zero. Edith was in France for a speaking engagement. Dr. Maples was on call. I had been told to phone in immediately if I ran a fever of more than 100. I was having dinner at my friend Kim Sadler's house.

"You don't look so good, Sunshine," she said with a frown. She insisted on taking my temperature.

"It's 102°, almost 103°. Call the doctor," she said.

I dialed the number to page Dr. Maples. He called back in minutes.

"You need to come to St. Luke's right away, Donna," he said.

"But I have to go back to work in a few minutes, Doc."

"Not tonight, you don't," he ordered. "Your body is totally defenseless. If you have an infection and we don't get it under control right away, you could die."

I spent the entire week in the hospital. Cooling blankets to control my fever, which approached 105°. Three IVs with different antibiotics in a desperate search to find out what was causing the fever. Finally, the doctors determined I had pneumonia. The drugs worked. My blood counts eventually recovered. We started again.

That's chemo.

I wanted desperately to move through these treatments, but the flashback served to temper my response.

"OK Edith, how long do you think we will have to wait?"

"Hopefully, just this week," she said. "We'll have to check the numbers again in a few days."

A few days later, they were still too low. My head was already adding the extra weeks onto the end of my chemo schedule. I wanted to be finished by Danielle's birthday, September 2nd.

"That would be a great birthday present, Mommy," she told me.

I knew from the beginning it was probably a pipe dream. One that was now a statistical impossibility.

"Sorry, baby doll," I thought, tears spilling down my face.

At least I was nearing the end of my radiation. That was something.

I wouldn't have to leave the kids every morning to get zapped.

Donna's Journal
Home > Health
June 18, 2002

Hi friends!
It's been quite a week since I last wrote. Your e-mails have truly been an inspiration. After hearing some of your stories... I feel like what I have to face is certainly surmountable.

I remember the first time I was diagnosed, I was amazed at the strong women and men who made me feel blessed to be a part of their struggle. I feel that way today. Some of you should also be stand up comedians! And there are at least a few of you whom, I believe, would be excellent choices to negotiate my next contract! You know I always try to get through things with humor. I don't know any other way... but I want you all to know you are in my heart and I appreciate you so much.

This is my last week of radiation...YEEEEAHH! Still a ways to go with the chemo... but hey we take 'em one hurdle at a time. As one of my dear friends reminds me frequently... every day's a gift.

God bless,
Donna

The friend I was referring to is Susan Mehrlust. A long time survivor of metastatic breast cancer, she beats the odds every day. She is in love with life, and ends every conversation with those words "every day's a gift." She doesn't just say them, she lives them. Susan breathes life into every moment. This is a woman who virtually lives on chemotherapy. She is utterly amazing. She left me messages all the time during my treatment. Not once did she take it personally if I didn't call her back.

The long hallway to radiation was shorter than usual. My stay in the waiting room less weighty. When I was called back to change, I wasn't counting clicks and buzzes in my head. This was finally it.

"Graduation day for you, right?"

I emerged from the stall in my white robe to see one of my cell mates in the dressing room.

"Hi," I smiled. "Yep, last one. How about you?"

"I'm just past half way, girl, but I'm getting there."

"It's good timing for me," I said. "This burn on my chest is starting to get gross."

There is no modesty between women going through cancer. I lifted my robe to show her the shredded, weeping red skin.

"That's nasty," she said. "Thanks for sharing. I guess that's what I have to look forward to."

No tasseled cap, no pomp and circumstance. But I was happier to graduate from radiation than I was to get my F.S.U. diploma.

"You hung tough," said Doctor Collie.

The game on his turf was over.

Break.

"I think your blood counts may be better now, without the radiation," Edith offered later on the phone. She was hopeful we could get back to a consistent chemo schedule. I was supposed to be three weeks on, one week off. I had only gotten through the first full cycle before we had to stop. There were five more cycles ahead.

"You know me, Edith," I joked. "The problem child."

I should have felt better. But I was so tired. The one-two punch of the chemo and radiation took its toll. I couldn't run anymore. I had injured myself just before this new madness started so even if I had the energy, running was out. Running is a drug for me. It helps me physically, and mentally it clears the cobwebs. I went to the gym and I rode my bike next to Tim while he ran everyday. It was something. But I resented him for having two strong legs and a healthy body.

The weather didn't help. That entire week it had poured and poured. Record rains. The gray skies matched my mood, and of course, they were Tim's fault too.

"Remember what Harold MacDonald used to say about running?" I asked Tim.

Harold used to work at the television station.

"He didn't like it right?"

"Well, he did it, but he never got that runner's high most of us get addicted to. He always accused me of stealing his endorphins."

"Now I'm stealing yours," Tim said.

"It's just hard to watch you do the things I want so desperately to do. Makes me feel like I'm sick or something." I smiled weakly.

Both times we caught the cancer before it ever made me feel sick. I tease Edith that I was never ill a day in my life until she got a hold of me.

"While we're talking endorphins, how's Frankel's Ironman training going?" Tim asked.

My friend Jon was preparing to do the Ironman competition in Hawaii. It's a concept that's tough to fathom even for those who love endurance sports.

A 2.4 mile swim, followed by a 112 mile bike. The final stage is a marathon - 26.2 miles.

"I don't know," I said. "I'll find out."

To: JonFrankel
Subject: Ironman

Hey there Jon boy,

Just wanted to check in and say hi. We've had a month's worth of rain in about two days. I think it's weighing on my psyche. One bright spot, I did finish my radiation today. Just chemo left. I so miss my physical strength... although I have been able to work out in some way or another most every day. Not like I'm used to. I decided on the long wig, by the way. Brenda is enjoying her new role in television news... and at least so far the viewers have been kind to her. Well enough of my rambling. I'm living vicariously through your Ironman training so let me know how it's going when you can.
And please, for the love of God, don't cut your hair like Matt Lauer's.
Yours in wading boots,
Donna

The phone rang. I picked it up before I even had a chance to think. I wasn't answering it much these days.

"Hey, woman, how are you?" Frankel's voice on the other end.

"I'm crappy, how's your training coming?"

"Knees are killing me. I can't run, but the bike and swim are OK."

"Someone HAS informed you that there's a little marathon at the end of your swim and bike right?"

"I'll get there when I have to."

"Won't we all," I thought.

Donna's Journal

Home > Health
June 25, 2002

Hi folks!
I hope you've dried out from the monsoons and are ready to face the summer!

Beyond your many words of encouragement many of you have asked me for good reading materials about breast cancer. Let me say off the bat that I probably read too much. I think I have just enough information now to be dangerous. But for those of you who are fighting or know someone who is fighting this battle... there is a book that I just love. Rosie O'Donnell wrote it along with a doctor a couple of years ago when I was first diagnosed. It has a lot of good basic information... and it makes you laugh in spite of yourself. It's called *Bosom Buddies*. I find that laughter helps me so much.

I hope you are checking out the websites we are posting in the journal as well. There is excellent information and support to be found in them. Speaking of support, yours continues to be breathtaking. Blood counts permitting, this should be a chemo week for me so if I look a little green later in the week, don't adjust your set! Truly, I am doing great and you all make it easier to see the light at the end of the tunnel.

God bless and have a great week.
Donna

I tried to accentuate the positive in my journal entries. In truth, while the letters kept me from derailing, I often feared the light at the end of the tunnel was really an oncoming train.

FOUR

Thank Heaven for Little Girls

To: donnahicken@firstcoastnews.com
Subject: Donna's Journal

hi-
I have never known any news reporters. But even if I had
I don't think any of them would have been as tuff as you.
I am 9 years old I attend Christ the King Catholic School.
My 14 year-old-sister will be attending Bishop Kenny High
School this fall. I read your diary page for the first time
today and I think you are tuff. I know you will pull through
just fine because you are a good person that is why God
would not want you to stay like this.
God Bless YOU
-Kallie-

I sat at my desk staring at this e-mail from a nine year old girl
and I buried my head in my hands. I was moved. I also felt like a
big fat fake.

"Oh, Kallie, I am SO NOT tough," I sighed.

I was overwrought, exhausted. I lost my focus on that "one
step." The race was already too long, and I was only beginning!
We were heading into the July ratings period and I felt tremendous
pressure to hang in there.

"Whatever you need, champ," my boss said. But that made me

53

feel worse.

"They aren't even counting on me," I thought.

But Mike couldn't win. If he asked me to do an extra show I was equally upset.

Doesn't anyone realize I'm just NOT up to this right now!

I wanted to work. I wanted to stay home. I wanted people to treat me like normal. I wanted to be babied. The invasion was complete. Somehow the faith of a nine year old child helped get me through the day.

Kallie Longley's Story
by Daniel J. Ovshak

Kallie Longley's first keyboard contact turned out to be a needed pep talk for one and a surprising reply for the other.

In 2002, the nine-year-old spent the summer with her grandmother, Elizabeth Stanczyk. It was a bonding time for the two. Kallie was the third generation to be raised in Jacksonville and her grandmother had stories to tell and Kallie had time to listen.

Kallie's favorite pastime was playing on-line computer games at the Disney and Nickelodeon Web sites. One afternoon while she was patiently waiting for her grandmother to finish up on the computer, Kallie noticed her grandmother was reading a letter with a picture of Donna Hicken in the corner.

Over her shoulder Kallie began reading about cancer, radiation and chemo. The computer games were forgotten for the moment. Kallie and her grandmother read the journal together. They read Donna's words from her heart.

For Kallie all of this was coming from the lady on the news. The lady who told them every day about other people. She told them sad stories, happy stories and stories that Kallie didn't always understand.

But that summer afternoon they were reading about the news

lady. They didn't stop there. Together they read Donna's journal entry from all the prior weeks. It became their ritual.

They looked forward to the next entry, hoping it would be one of encouragement and good news. This was a whole new world for Kallie, following the entries of a local celebrity, a news anchor, facing a serious health challenge.

"I thought it would be fun to write to Donna, to see how she was doing. Her journal was the best thing I'd ever read," said Kallie.

Her grandmother, Mrs. Stanczyk, reviewed the e-mail before it was sent and only had one criticism. "I told her that the proper spelling was t-o-u-g-h, not tuff. But Kallie insisted that she wanted to spell it TUFF."

"I didn't think she'd write me because I'd never done e-mail before," said Kallie. "I didn't think she'd have time to write back. But Donna wrote to me within an hour. She told me she was doing fine and she was trying the best she could to get through this."

Kallie lives with her mother, Leslie Stanczyk and her fifteen year old sister Katie in an Arlington town home. Though Katie is older, she still finds time to play kickball and go to the movies with Kallie. "It didn't surprise me at all when Kallie wrote to Donna. She's always been a very caring child. I would have been surprised if she hadn't written," her mother said.

"Kallie and Katie are like day and night. Now that Katie is a teenager, her interests lean towards driving and boys," said Leslie. "But they both love music; Katie listening to her own special choices and Kallie making it," Mrs. Stanczyk said.

Kallie is interested in all the Arts. She loves singing, dancing, acting and playing the piano. If she doesn't do it, she just hasn't tried it yet. Most of us can remember that special moment when we picked up our first musical instrument or sang our first song. Kallie has no memory of not singing, dancing or playing the piano. "I've just always done it," she smiles.

She has her future figured out. She even has a backup plan. "I'd like to be an actress or singer, but if that doesn't work out I'd like to go to the University of Florida and be a pediatrician," Kallie said.

Kallie found she had common ground with Donna. "She told me that she went to Bishop Kenny, and that's where my sister goes, too!"

Reading how Donna's week was going became a big part of Kallie's week. "I read her journal, and she wrote about everything she had done," Kallie said.

One of the biggest surprises for Kallie was when Donna decided to start wearing her wigs. "I thought it was really really sad. I thought Donna cut her hair because she wanted to. She said that a lot of people didn't like the way she looked. I thought she still looked pretty," said Kallie.

This was Kallie's first encounter with someone fighting a disease. "I don't know anyone personally who has cancer, but my great-grandmother had brain cancer. I was a baby when she died, so I didn't really know her. She's the only person, other than Donna, that I know of with cancer," Kallie said.

An avid reader of mysteries, Kallie also loves Harry Potter books and movies. Action packed 'Charlie's Angels' is also high on her list. Not surprising considering how TUFF they are. As for real life heroes, Kallie is still a little surprised at the friendship she's developed with Donna. "I've e-mailed her three times and she's answered every time. It was amazing because Donna is very busy and has so many people that want to talk to her. She has so many people supporting her," said Kallie.

People have asked Kallie if she's given Donna any advice. "No. She's one of the toughest people I know, so I don't think there's anything I could tell her. She really had to be strong and she had to put her faith in God, because nothing can happen without Him. God is who everyone needs and Donna really hung in there."

Kallie's voice softens, "I thought Donna had to be very strong, to like, endure what she went through," she sighed. "It had to be very painful."

Donna's Journal
Home > Health
July 2, 2002

Hi friends...
I got a letter from a nine year old girl today named Kallie. She says I am "tuff." I told her I do my best... but I have to admit I feel a little guilty. I really wasn't that tough last week. On the whine scale from one to ten... I think I scored about an 11. It happens. My upper lip sometimes loses its stiffness. Sometimes I forget what normal feels like and it makes me sad. Kallie helped.

I did have a short term problem this week with my e-mail replies being returned to me... so if you asked me for a specific piece of advice or information and I didn't respond... please write back. It may just be that I haven't gotten there yet... but it may be that my computer was kerflooy.

Also lots of responses about cancer books. "It's Not About the Bike" by Lance Armstrong is also out of this world... worth a second... and third read.

And to those of you who have written me about friends who are having trouble with treatment because of costs... I assure you I am making this a mission. That is simply unacceptable. I'll be sharing some plans with you soon. Stay tuned!
Can you tell I'm feeling a little emotional this week? Sorry if I've rambled. Thanks for sticking with me and have a great week.

God bless,
Donna

To: donnahicken@firstcoastnews.com
Subject: Drew's Friend

Dear Ms. Hicken,
My name is Jennifer Ronzon. I go to school with Drew.
When I found out you were sick, I told Drew I felt bad for
your family.
I have a disease too. I know how it is to have to go to
doctors all the time. I also get tired all the time.
Get better soon,
Jennifer Ronzon

To: JenniferR
Subject: RE: Drew's Friend

Hi Jennifer!
You are so sweet to write to me. I'm glad Drew goes to
school with someone who is so thoughtful. We are doing
well getting through this together... I hope and pray you
are doing well also. God bless and thanks again for the
nice words.
Donna

To: donnahicken@firstcoastnews.com
Subject: Courage

Donna,
You have been there for others during their times of need.
Through all the rough times in our lives, you have offered
information and support by being there as a beacon of
light. But I write you today not asking you to give of
yourself but rather asking you to receive. Though I am
also a cancer survivor, I am not asking you for your advice,
although I am sure it would be very informative. Nor do I

write to you asking for books or treatments that you think might help me or others I know battle this foe. Today I write to you, Donna, to uplift you and to provide encouragement to you as you yourself fight your battle.

I only wish that we could somehow return unto you the blessing you have been to us. Your courage has been a source of strength for so many. I will never forget the Sunday after the Gate River Run when, rather than displaying the photo of the man who won the race, there... in living color... Donna Hicken embraces another hairless race finisher... and mere days since completing chemotherapy. I found it very fitting since your race was indeed the greatest victory!!

Day after day, your courage to go on with life, wimpy upper lip and all, serves to remind us all that we live each day as it comes. Perhaps whining, with wig on head.... but always there, taking each day as it comes. You are allowed to whine, to be human and to cry. I learned through my own battle that for these things there is no language but a cry. There are so many who stand with you Donna. Your name surfaces in almost every conversation I am involved in on the subject of cancer. And, since I believe in the power of prayer, I say one for you each time.

Though none of us are guaranteed tomorrow, your continued valiant fight provides hope for those who continue to fight. I don't know why you have been stricken and would never wish it on anyone. However, since it has happened, I am grateful that you chose to allow others to share in your suffering with you, and to use your calling to the public eye to educate others. You and Jeannie have done so much to heighten the awareness of cancer in our area and beyond. I will always be grateful to you for your willingness to allow us to share with you.

I am fortunate in that *Road Runner Sports* published my story in their most recent book, "Running for the Woman's Soul." I found out in February. Yesterday I received my complimentary copy and felt honored that I could perhaps encourage others to run and to overcome cancer. Today I saw you on the 5:30 news and felt disappointment rise within me. Rather than my story being published, I wished the space had been used to share YOUR story. You are a courageous warrior and your story would have made so much more of an impact. You are a heroine, Donna.
May God Bless and keep you until you are totally restored to perfect health.
Reba J. Hoffman

To: RebaHoffman
Subject: RE: Courage

Dear Reba,
What a beautiful letter. I'm the one who is truly blessed by the friendship and caring of people like you. Thank you so much for your kind words. They mean more to me than I could ever express. God bless.
Donna

The e-mails massaged my aching psyche. But there was something else that was slowly but surely taking up more space in my brain. Letters, and phone calls from people who were in my same boat, but didn't have a good job, or insurance or support. Most of the time, they weren't even asking for money. They just wanted someone to listen, or pray.

"I don't have the luxury to worry if I will be here for my son," one woman sobbed into the phone. "I don't even know if I'll be able to feed him after this week."

I listened. I tried to help. Mostly, I felt a deep sense of frustration that any woman should have to face a deadly disease and worry about feeding her kids. Back when I was first diagnosed, I set my mind on starting a foundation for women living with breast cancer who had financial troubles.

My friend Robin had lost her Medicaid because her husband's truck broke down and he had to buy another one.

"But it's a used truck," she begged the woman at the Medicaid office, "and he has to have it for his construction job."

Robin is a pistol. She says it like it is. She and Glenn have five kids and they both work their tails off to support them. Like so many people, they let their insurance lapse during a particularly tough financial month and of course that's when she got the diagnosis. The treatment she received from both the medical community and the government was appalling.

"You'll be lucky if I treat you," one doctor told her, his picture of Jesus on the wall behind him. "I'm not going to make a dime."

This was while her Medicaid was still intact. After the truck incident, Robin couldn't complete her reconstructive surgery, and couldn't get her follow-up medications.

"If I don't take that medicine, my cancer might come back and I could die," she explained to the woman at the Medicaid office.

"I guess you should have thought about that before you had five children," the clerk shot back.

The story made me livid. I wanted to do something, but I never followed through.

This time I couldn't fail. "I have to get this done," I told Tim that night. "Here I am, getting showered with all this love and support. I have to find a way to give it back to people."

"You will, Donna," he said. "Just get through your chemo and you can put all your energy into it."

That was Tim's way of telling me not to bite off more than I

61

could chew.

Meantime, word of my plan started to make its way through the grapevine. I was already getting offers for help.

To: Hicken, Donna
Subject: Cancer Foundation

Donna —
Donna LePre e-mailed you about my ad agency. We will be glad to help you at no cost with anything you need to launch your efforts. Please let me clarify that I had throat/thyroid cancer and not breast cancer. My cancer spread and affected both breasts and my left shoulder, but it was not technically breast cancer. Just wanted to set the record straight. Please call me if I can be of service to you. I praise God for the opportunity to help.
Cynthia Montello

To: CynthiaMontello
Subject: RE: Cancer Foundation

Wow... thanks Cynthia!
I will definitely take you up on your offer. I am just starting to get the paperwork together... it was a lot more stuff than I thought... but when I get set up I'm going to let you know. I'm really excited about it. The need is so great. If you have any ideas I'd love to hear them. Thanks again for your interest... and I'll definitely be getting in touch.
Donna

I had already contacted our friend Steve Prom. Steve is a lawyer and has done a lot of foundation work in the past. He e-mailed me the set-up paperwork at the speed of light. I took one look at it and was totally overwhelmed. I couldn't even figure out how to open half the attachments.

But it was a start.

Donna's Journal
Home > Health
July 15, 2002

Hello...

I have to start out this week's journal entry with a confession.

I am practically illiterate when it comes to using my computer! I've known this for some time now... but it was confirmed for me once and for all last week. I have assumed that when you write to me on the "discussion boards" that those entries go to my e-mail. Therefore I have been responding only to my e-mail and not to the discussion boards. Our wonderful webmaster had explained this to me... however in my computer phobic brain it did not compute. I will get it together one of these days... and by then the computers will change and I'll have to start over!! I blame "Brenda." For those of you just joining me... that is the name I have affectionately given to my wig.

No chemo last week... so I feel pretty good. Back to the grind this week, blood counts permitting. No chemo weeks are so great. Food starts to taste like... well... food... and I have the energy to keep up with my Tasmanian devil (my 7-year-old son). The kids are so terrific through this. My son... in his best announcer

63

voice...makes fun of my bald head. "Hey isn't that Donna Hicken from the news...why she's bald... that's just a shame." All this as he giggles himself into a stomach ache. My daughter (who I believe was born 40 like me) can only roll her eyes and wonder what planet brought him to us.

I'd better stop before they get mad at me. As always thank you for your continued support. I couldn't ask for better. Have a great week!!

Your master of megabytes,
Donna

To: donnahicken@firstcoastnews.com
Subject: Record news partner checks in

Hi Donna,
I am pleased that your spirits are so up and that you still have that infectious laugh in spite of all that you are going through. I have been keeping you in my prayers having felt as though we were bonded in several respects, journalists and breast cancer survivors about six months apart; July 5, 2000.
We were on the same panel for EPIC last December at St. Johns River CC but were not introduced.
I enjoyed your column this week on your son's response to your bald head. Mine, then 22 when I went through chemo, used to come home from college and ask me to let him "check the fuzz." He offered a couple of times to shave it smooth for me telling me it would grow faster. I declined his offer. But the bond we have today is much stronger because of what we went through together. He would call home and talk to his father and ask him

questions about the status of my treatments. Then, after a time, he would talk to me and not ask any questions but only tell funny stories about bald people. Alas, he is in grad school at that school in Tallahassee, shunning my alma mater in Gainesville now twice. I e-mailed him tonight and told him to read your column of the 15th.
Continued best wishes,
Margo C. Pope
Associate Editor
The St. Augustine Record

To: MargoPope
Subject: RE: Record news partner checks in

Hi Margo!
Thanks so much for taking the time to read the journal....and beyond that for spending the energy to write. I enjoyed your comments that day at the college and of course I know you by your wonderful work. I'm glad to hear your cancer brought you closer to your son. I always hope it does that for us.... but sometimes I worry that they get sick of the sickness. They really are just great kids. Sounds like you beat your cancer and are doing well. (Aside from the sheer embarrassment of having your child in enemy territory!) My Danielle, I'm afraid, is leaning toward the orange and blue... but Drew is still firmly entrenched in garnett and gold. Well I suppose I should get some work done. Thanks again for taking the time. Continued good health to you and God bless.
Donna

I admit it. I hate computers. I was the last person in the newsroom to receive mine because I insisted on keeping my old clickity-click typewriter as long as possible. I finally gave it up, kicking and screaming all the way, but beyond logging on, and getting my stories filed for the news, I don't care to know another thing. I know this is immature. I don't care.

"Wow Donna, amazing what's coming in on the discussion boards about you." I turned in my chair to see our webmaster. "Are you going to start writing back soon?"

I gave Thomas a blank look. "I write back to just about everybody, or at least I try," I said.

My blank look was returned.

Turns out, I was responding to e-mails, which I thought were somehow connected to the discussion boards.

"I'm an idiot, OK?" I said.

Thomas smiled though I'm sure inside he was thinking the same thing.

We got it straightened out although I would have relapses into stupidity.

To: Wilson, Thomas
Subject: I'm Pathetic

Thomas, once again I have tried and tried and I can't seem to make the reply work on the discussion board. It keeps telling me I have an incorrect login... please help the stupid at your earliest opportunity.
Donna

Interesting thing discussion boards. Here I was having personal conversations that everyone could read. It's sort of voyeuristic, isn't it? People were great, but it was hard for me to engage. What I told myself was that these discussions helped more people. Not just me and the person writing to me. But I was far more likely to have a heart-to-heart on e-mail.

"No chemo this week, Hicken?" my 11p.m. co-anchor, Alan

Gionet, popped his head over my cubicle wall.

"Nope, another reprieve," I said. "Blood counts are still too puny."

I think Alan appreciated no chemo weeks almost as much as I did.

He could sit at his desk, the cubicle next to mine, and eat his blue cheese, double deluxe, dripping with fat cheeseburger without fear that I would throw up.

"You seem like you're feeling pretty good," he said. "How are the kids?"

"They're great," I said. "I think Drew is going to be a stand-up comedian when he grows up. That is unless Danielle kills him first."

Alan laughed. He loves to talk about his kids and seems to enjoy talking about anyone else's just as much.

And my kids were doing great. I was so thankful for that. Out of everyone in my life they treated me most like me through all this. Sometimes when I was with them, I could almost forget.

Donna's Journal
Home > Health
July 22, 2002

Hello friends!

I'm feeling very energetic this week. The reason...no chemo. If you read last week's journal you know that wasn't the plan. Unfortunately my blood counts didn't cooperate and consequently I have an extra week "off".

It's sort of a double edged sword... this not having chemo. I feel as close to normal this week as I have since I started the process.

For instance... this week... bread doesn't taste like metal. I'm not craving red meat (something I rarely eat normally... but seem to need during treatment). I'm exercising almost as much as I want. Generally, even with puny blood counts, my body is singing a happy tune.

Then there's my brain. It works on me. Am I getting enough medicine into my body to fight this monster... is it enough to finally end this invasion of my life once and for all? How much of the Jekyll and Hyde can my kids take... or the people I love? I can drive myself crazy. My doctor should get paid double for all the questions I ask.

The bottom line is... I'm doing what I can do. I can't have chemo while my blood counts are down... I can't answer any of those questions about life in a definitive way. So I find myself back to where I started... where all of us go when we realize we don't have control over our own lives and that we never did. I look up... and I say thanks for the gift of today.

I want to thank all of you who continue to share your own stories with me. I know you can relate. We are all here to serve each other. I hope I help you a fraction of how you've helped me.

Have a good week and God bless,
Donna

"And she's making this climb in the Pyrenees like it's nothing, ladies and gentlemen. She's mano a mano with the mountain. This woman isn't human," I feigned the voice of the announcer from the Tour de France. Tim was running beside me laughing as I pedaled my beach cruiser up a small incline in Atlantic Beach.

"Come on, surfer boy," I teased. "Is that all you got?"

During chemo weeks, if I could turn the pedals on my bike at all, it was a victory. Now, we were coming up on three weeks since my last treatment. My blood counts just weren't holding the way Edith had hoped after radiation. She was hesitant to start me on blood boosters this early in the game, but she was about to give in. A drug called GCSF (Granulocyte Colony Stimulating Factor) would pump up my white counts and make it possible for me to be treated. It has its drawbacks. Among them, terrible bone pain as the marrow struggles to produce, and shots every day.

"Strong ride today, young lady," Tim said.

"Yeah, Lance better watch his back," I smiled. Tim and I never missed a day of the Tour de France. The sight of Lance Armstrong "dancing" up the mountains made me feel like superwoman. Here's this guy, who has virtually no chance of surviving cancer. He battles back on what seems like pure will and goes on to dominate the field in cycling year in and year out. He's every cancer patient's dream. If Lance can do it, so can I.

"I think I'll go to the gym today," I said.

"Wow, the bike and the gym, you ARE feeling good."

"I am, but the energy is also driving me a little crazy. It's just postponing the inevitable. And how do I know this is even helping me beat the cancer?"

"You just have to trust Edith," Tim said.

"It's not like I have a choice," I muttered.

I did trust Edith, but I hated not knowing what was going on inside my body. I was sick of the delays.

"Haven't I been patient enough?" I thought.

"Patience" is not a word in my vocabulary. I am as type "A" as it gets. I want it done now, and I want it done right (which means my way), and I don't want to hear any excuses.

Most of all, I want control. I had none at the moment, and the worst part was, I was realizing, I never did. I knew this intellectually just the way people know intellectually they are going to die one day. But no one believes it. Not really. I didn't either until someone told me I had cancer.

FIVE

Potato Salad and Other Comfort Food

It took a few minutes for the room to come into focus. When it did, it started to spin. Up off the bed, into the bathroom, head in the toilet. Just in time. Welcome back to chemo.

"If I have to throw up there should at least be alcohol involved," I murmured to myself.

My tongue felt like it was growing hair. My head was a dull hazy ache. I looked up to see my image in the mirror.

"Just another day in paradise," I said to the bald red-eyed alien staring back at me.

"Moooooooomy!" I heard Danielle's voice down the hall. That sing-songy way she says my name when I know she's about to tell on her brother. "Drew's got your wig on."

Andrew came running down the hall, giggling like he'd just told the funniest joke ever. Danielle was right behind. She was not amused.

I love my son's giggle. It heals me. One time he left a message on my cell phone and I saved it for weeks just to hear him laugh.

Drew screeched to a stop in front of me, put his hands through the long blonde locks, and cocked his head.

"Very pretty, dontcha think?"

"Mommy, I told him you need that for work and not to touch it," Danielle said. My little protector.

"Did NOT," Drew returned.

"It's all right," I said. "I actually don't need Brenda anymore. I got a new wig. One without bangs."

"What are you going to call her, Mommy?" Danielle asked.

"Jennifer."

"Why Jennifer?"

"I wasn't very creative this time. Jennifer was the name on the box. I guess they name all those wigs. Go figure. Mommy's not the only silly one."

"So I can really have the wig?" Drew asked.

"Yes, Drewina daaaahling, I think you look stunning."

Drew giggled, stuck his tongue out at Danielle and ran back down the hall.

"He's so weird," Danielle said shaking her head.

"Come give me a hug Miss Pooh," I said, stretching my arms out. "You may as well know it now, all men are."

I was still replaying the scene in my head that afternoon as I drove into work. I smiled at the thought of how easy it was for them to just be. To them I was Mommy, not a cancer patient, or a bald wonder.

I thought about my words to Danielle. While I was teasing, I knew there would be a day she would find out for herself about that crazy dance between women and men. How we all try to understand each other. The frustrations of it and the joys.

"Please let me be here to see it Lord," I prayed.

The tears came so fast and hard that I had to sit in the car for a while before I could compose myself enough to walk into the station.

"Don't go there, Donna," I told myself. "Don't even go there."

I logged on to my computer to get my daily dose of courage, and the first letter held me transfixed.

A woman named Kathy wrote to commend me for my courage under fire. She then confided that her own sweet seven-year-old son had passed away a few months earlier after battling cancer for four years. She said his kind, fun loving spirit throughout the ordeal reminded her of me and that she got great comfort out of picturing her son helping Jesus give me the strength I need.

MY courage under fire?

72

"Jesus, Mary and Joseph," I said as the tears came again. "How does she live?"

I cried so long at the thought of this woman's compassion and courage that I had to put ice on my face before I could deliver the news. I still got a number of phone calls from people "hoping Donna's OK."

It was a full two days later when I finally mustered enough courage to write back.

To: Kathy
Subject: So sorry

Dear Kathy,
How lovely of you to spend the energy to write me considering your own devastating loss. I am so sorry... sorry beyond words. I can't imagine anything more difficult than losing a child. The thought of him with Jesus is the most inspirational comfort. Thank you so much for thinking of me... for praying for me. I will pray for you as well. I'm sure your hurt is overwhelming. Thankfully so is the love of Christ. God bless you and hang in! Again thank you for being so thoughtful.
Donna

It is impossible to quantify what one letter like Kathy's did for me. "This woman gets it," I thought. "Be Jesus for others."

Would I have been unselfish enough to relive that kind of pain to help someone else get over theirs?

I wondered.

Probably not.

It was the week for such unselfish offerings.

To: donnahicken@firstcoastnews.com
Subject: Bear

Dear Ms. Hicken:
I need to complete my wife's wish so please let me take a few minutes of your time. My wife had colon cancer and breast cancer. She would always watch your news program and prayed for your continued health.
Her breast cancer came back in her lower back, hips, liver and lungs. During her last few weeks she would come in and out of consciousness. Once you were on TV and she commented that you had done your hair differently. I explained to her what happened and she stated "when I get better I am sending her my rainbow bear and I'll say an extra prayer for Donna." She then lapsed into her semiconscious state. Finally on June 8, 2002 she passed away after fighting for over 6 years.
I have the teddy bear that she wanted you to have and need to get it to you somehow, I realize that packages are difficult to deliver but at least I had to make an attempt to fulfill my wife's wish. I can take it in person or send my daughter or mail it. How ever it would be easier for you. Thank you for your time.
Sam Gil

Sam's letter was heartbreaking. I could feel him restraining his emotions as he wrote. How he could even part with that bear I couldn't fathom. How a woman so close to death herself, thought of comforting someone else was beyond me as well.

To: SamGil
Subject: Thank you

Dear Sam,
I'm so terribly sorry to hear that you've lost your sweet wife to this horrible disease. She sounds like a very loving

person. I hope her passing was peaceful. I don't try to understand why these things happen. I just trust that one day God will let me know. I will keep you in my prayers. I know you must be really hurting. I would be more than honored to have your wife's bear. How ever you wish to send it will be fine. I'd love to meet you if you come by the station. I hope this won't sound trite to you, but I do believe those we love become our guardian angels when they pass.. existing only slightly beyond the realm of our vision. God's peace and comfort be with you and I look forward to hearing from you soon.
Sincerely,
Donna

As I searched my heart for the right words to say to Sam, my mind went immediately to a dedication my Aunt Donna wrote and placed on the back of my cousin Michel's wedding invitation. Our family had recently lost a number of loved ones, including her mother and my father. Reading it, I could almost touch my sweet Daddy. I could feel his presence right there. Smell him, hear his powerful tenor voice. My aunt had the dedication framed for me on my birthday one year, and it still hangs in my home. I read it when I need to be with my Dad.

Dedicated to the presence of Angels
To those who live among us in everyday life,
and to those whose memories are engraved on the crevices of our
minds and exist only slightly beyond the realm of our vision:
We love you, we miss you, we learned so much from you,
And we are grateful.

The image of my father existing just out of my sight is such a comfort. I hoped Sam would feel the same.

Sam Gil's Story
by Oscar Senn

"I love potato salad," Sam Gil says with fondness.

Sam, a 54 year-old Social Studies teacher at Robert E. Lee High School, is affable and plainspoken. He wears a curling beard that shows some gray. When he talks of his late wife his eyes shine.

"Dianne made the best potato salad in the world. The best I've ever had in my life. If you want to know what kind of person Dianne was, I'll tell you about the recipe she gave me.

"In the last year of her illness she was pretty much bedridden. We were spending time together one day and she says to me, 'I want some potato salad. I wish I could get up and make us some.' I said, 'Well, you could tell me how to do it, and I could try to fix it.' She accepted the challenge and I shuttled back and forth from her to the kitchen, taking instructions. Her recipe is quite elaborate, it takes a couple of hours, but when I was through we were able to sit down and enjoy. It wasn't as good as hers, but I thought it was pretty good.

"I, of course, thought I was doing her a favor making the potato salad. I thought it was my idea. Well, a year or so after her death my daughter Beth said to me, 'Dinner tonight would be great with some of Mom's potato salad.' I said, 'Hey, I can do that. She taught me how to make it.' It was then I realized that was Dianne's plan all along. She led me every step of the way learning that recipe, so that we would still have her potato salad when she was gone. That's what she was like."

Dianne Gil's battle with cancer was a long and torturous one, lasting more than seven years. She was diagnosed with colon cancer in 1995.

Dianne started having problems a year earlier, complaining to her doctor about pain in her lower abdomen. She was passing blood, but kept that information private from Sam.

"She was in pain all the time," Sam remembers with justifiable anger.

"The doctor did test after test. He thought it might be gastroenteritis, and a whole bunch of other things I no longer remember. I tried to get her to complain, but she was very, very trusting. Finally after a whole year of tests he called in another doctor and that's when we found out about the cancer."

Dianne was slated to undergo a bowel resection with colostomy to remove two inches of colon when it ruptured, increasing the urgency of the operation.

"The night before the operation she was in severe pain all night long. We went to the hospital at 8:00 in the morning. She hurt so much, and they kept her standing up filling out forms. I complained, but they just kept saying they would take care of it with the operation. They operated at two in the afternoon and discovered her colon had ruptured."

What should have been a brief resection and colostomy ended up taking nearly three hours. The price-tag for the resulting two-week hospital convalescence was over $350,000, not counting subsequent rounds of chemotherapy.

"Granted we had insurance," Sam says, "but what happens to women who don't have insurance? Our finances really went downhill, even though we were covered for most of the things the doctors wanted to do."

After recuperating from the surgery, Dianne underwent fourteen months of extensive chemotherapy.

Sam recalls there were five different rounds of chemotherapy, but all the varied treatments and their nightmarish effects blur together.

"The medications that you take to deal with the side effects of the medications you're already taking," Sam says, shaking his head sadly. "She had 17 different drugs at one time. I had to take over her schedule because she couldn't remember when to take them anymore. I had boxes of pills with times written all over them and made lists, all kinds of stuff to help us remember."

There was also much prayer-therapy from Sam, Dianne, their family and home congregation. The combination of medicine and faith proved effective. Little more than a year after her surgery, the doctors cautiously announced victory.

"The colon cancer never bothered her again."

Sam and Dianne decided to take a much-needed holiday to one of their favorite places, Maine. It was a celebration of her surviving colon cancer.

"We always drove," Sam says, bemused. "Dianne was not an airplane person. I'd say, 'You know, for every day in the car, it's one hour in the air.' But she didn't care. We even talked about getting a Winnebago."

On the trip Dianne told Sam the doctors had discovered a lump in one breast during a routine follow-up examination.

"We had two weeks from the time they found the lump until they took it out. She was colon cancer free when they gave her the other tests and discovered the breast cancer. The chemo was over. Then they found the lump. The doctors at first thought it was benign, but it wasn't."

The new diagnosis of cancer came two weeks later. "Dianne and I only had two weeks together before the second diagnosis."

"That made two primary cancers," Sam remembers. "The primary colon cancer came first, and then it went away, then she had primary breast, which was not related to the other one. The breast cancer metastasized and went to the brain and the liver."

Dianne immediately started on a new regimen of medications, intensive chemotherapy to stop the breast cancer, and radiation to kill it.

"On top of all that the radiation treatment for the breast cancer started crumbling her upper vertebras. So she was in a neck brace for six months while she was having chemo for the breast cancer."

Sam throws up his hands. "I thought, 'How can somebody be

so unlucky?'" Cancer had already struck down his favorite aunt, Aunt Ruth, and his dearest cousin, Alina, as well as his best friend Wade.

"But to Dianne," Sam says, "it was all part of God's plan. She never for a single instant saw it as punishment, but she fought it every step of the way."

"One time I asked her, 'Did you ever ask God, 'Why me?' and she got really indignant. She considered death to be the beginning of her life with God.

"She fought the cancer all the way to the end. I gave up sometimes. It was painful to see somebody in so much pain. Especially since she was so brave. I only heard her cry out one time, and that was when they gave her the spinal tap. And I think if the doctor had told her she would have never cried out. It was one of those unexpected things.

"She definitely didn't like being under medication. I felt bad about putting the patch on her, but I said I'm sorry, but I'm not going to see you die in pain. If you're going to die, you're going to die comfortable."

One time I prayed, "God, if you're going to take her, please take her. Why drag this out any more?"

"It was hard for me to understand why she had so much pain. Because there was a lot of pain. But if you go to church, just about every church has two or three sermons about 'Why do good things happen to bad people and bad things happen to good people.' Dianne just thought, 'This is the way this is supposed to be,' and that was the way it was for her. She said, 'I'm just here. Whenever He wants to call on me to leave, I'm ready.'"

Dianne Gil believed there was a plan for her life, and that her long struggle with cancer was part of that plan. "You know that book, 'God is my Co-Pilot'?" Sam says. "Well, Dianne used to say, 'God's the pilot. I'm just the co-pilot.' She didn't complain about anything."

Sam and Dianne Gil were married in 1971, but their story begins much earlier. They started dating in Junior High School, in Naples, Florida. When Sam joined the army and was stationed in Germany, Dianne was the only girl he kept in touch with. He resumed their courtship on his return, and they married not long afterward. Dianne gave birth to their son Steven in 1973 and daughter Beth came along in 1975.

Sam smiles when he talks about Dianne in those days. "She was skinny and tall. Six feet, a little taller than I was, and skinnier than me. She had millions of freckles. Her wrists were about that big around. She was a tiny thing." Sam makes an "O" with his thumb and forefinger.

His eyes sparkle, his voice slows. "But, I'll tell you, her greatest attribute was her sense of humor. She could find humor in any situation. Sometimes she would laugh at things I didn't think were funny.

"She always wanted to go to Dollywood, in Nashville. Well, we went there and I was pushing her around in her wheelchair. That place is hilly, and I had to work pretty hard. She looked at me and said, 'I may have cancer, but you're the one sweating.' Things like that. She would joke about her illness and the doctors. She could laugh about all of it."

"Amazing Grace" was their song. "We'd get mad at each other, and she'd be cleaning the house. And I would start humming that song and she would start singing it in the other room without even hearing me. It was weird. And after that our fight was over. So that became our song. It was played at her funeral. She loved it."

It was a bear that connects him with Donna Hicken. He and Dianne liked to visit State Parks and especially loved the Smoky Mountains. A favorite hike was Cade's Cove in Tennessee, where the deer walk right up to you, and bears make frequent appearances. Dianne began collecting bears.

She had bear magnets and bear pendants and several stuffed Teddy Bears of different sizes and personalities. Shortly after beginning her first round of chemo, Dianne got an addition to her collection.

It was a little brown fellow, arms open wide as if waiting for a hug. He was chubby and smiling. He wears a card reminding, "Faith Changes Rainclouds Into Rainbows." She was given the bear by a fellow teacher at Mandarin Oaks Elementary during her first hospital stay.

The bear became a constant companion during Dianne's illness, a mascot. For six years he stood vigil at her bedside. He sat patiently in waiting rooms, and, on subsequent hospital stays Sam would bring the bear for visits.

"I think the bear reminded her of the mountains. She loved hiking. That was the hardest part for her, not being outdoors. I saw her regress from using a walking stick, to a cane, to a four-pointed cane, to a walker, to a wheelchair, to a wheelchair with oxygen. It was very hard."

Her last time home from the hospital Dianne was very sick. She was on multiple medications, and went in and out of awareness of her surroundings. When Sam and Dianne watched TV she sat in a big comfortable green chair in the den, her oxygen bottle nearby. Channel 12 was their local news station.

"We thought that program was friendly. Dianne liked to watch Donna," Sam remembers.

One night Dianne said, "What's wrong with Donna? Why is she wearing her hair like that?"

Sam explained that the newscasters breast cancer had come back, and she was going through chemotherapy. That was why she wore a wig.

Dianne took the news thoughtfully. When Donna's segment ended she said, "I'm going to give my bear to Donna so she can get well."

And then she went to sleep.

Dianne died a month before she would have turned 53, June 8, 2002.

"The telephone rings and then you die," Sam says. It was what he used to say to his kids, to explain the arbitrary nature of human life.

"They would come to me and say, 'Dad, that's not fair.' And I would say, 'Life's not fair. The telephone rings and then you die.' It can be any time. I just made that up, to tell them how unfair life could be. And it happened to her. Because the telephone rang, and it was our son from the U.S. Kennedy.

"Steven fortunately was able to come from the Kennedy when she was first in the hospital. They flew him from the Persian Gulf. And when he left then it was very difficult, knowing that he might be saying goodbye for the last time.

"He said, 'Dad, I just decided to call'. It takes twenty minutes for them to route the call from the carrier."

"'She's here,' I said, 'do you want to say hello or goodbye?' So I put the phone on the pillow by her head. I don't know what he said to her.

"And she died literally less than three minutes later. I was right outside and I just turned around. I didn't want to see it. You could hear her breathing coming very hard. I heard my cousin Alina's last breath, and I didn't want to hear Dianne's."

Dianne saw her illness as part of God's plan. "The way it brought people together. She had a very big family, and we have sort of small nuclear family. It united everybody. Our son and daughter started coming by much more often, and her family made frequent trips from Naples. When I heard about Donna's work and the Journal, the e-mails and all, I thought about what Dianne always said. Maybe it's His plan to bring us all closer together."

*   *   *

I arrived at work one day to find Dianne Gil's rainbow bear on my desk. I gave it a long squeeze.

"God bless you Dianne," I said.

Sam and I never met. The bear lives in my room.

82

Donna's Journal
Home > Health
July 29, 2002

Hello friends...

So many thoughts this week. I'll start with you. It's rare that I will go somewhere... or open an e-mail, etc. that someone doesn't stop and offer an encouraging word. One which usually includes a thank you for sharing my experience. It's very nice... but the truth is I think it helps me more than anyone else.

Just a couple of examples. I received an e-mail from a mom last week... after I wrote about my crazy seven-year-old and his great attitude about all of this. She doesn't have her seven-year-old anymore. He died recently from cancer. I could certainly feel her sadness... but she told me it gives her comfort to think of her own fun-loving son helping Jesus to give me strength. Wow.

Then there was the sweet gentleman who struggled to write to me about the recent death of his wife to cancer. Every night she held her rainbow bear... and it was her final wish that I receive it for strength.
There are so many more. The thing that jumps out at me with all of the stories I hear is that people are hopeful. Yes they are sad... and they wish things could be different... but they still do their best to stay positive and help others. I find that tremendously inspirational.

I'm not usually one to post notes to myself... or depend on certain phrases to lift me... but there is one in the clinic that always sticks with me. "Life is 10% what happens to you... and 90% your attitude about it." I like it.

OK... on a practical note... for all of you who are wondering... yes Brenda is taking a break... I now have Jennifer... hope you like her... I was having trouble seeing through the bangs.

I had chemo this week... so we're back on track for the moment... and I'll be taking a few days off next week... but not to worry... just for fun.

Have a great week and God bless,

Donna

The days off were for my wedding.

"Today's your father's birthday, isn't it?" Tim asked.

"Yes, August 1st. I wish he was going to be here to see us get married."

"He'll see us," Tim said, squeezing my shoulders.

My father was in my thoughts more and more these days. Every now and then I would even get a note from someone who knew and loved him. People would often comment on his courage as he faced a lifetime of illness.

"You get it from him," they'd say, and it made my chest rise.

My dad got sick at the exact same age as me, 38. He had kidney failure. He was a lawyer, but at one time had a promising career as an opera singer.

I remember proudly showing his souvenir from the Metropolitan Opera in New York at my fifth grade show and tell.

"My dad was a runner-up at the Met," I bragged. I still do.

He would sing to me all the time and in my head he still does.

My dad and I were inseparable. Literally. When I was 19, I gave him a kidney. Years of dialysis had taken a horrible toll. My mom cried all the way to the hospital. I never gave it a second thought. The only thought I couldn't stand was living without him.

"You look funny," I said to him as they wheeled us past each other on the way to the operating room. We were both wearing those puffy blue surgical caps.

"See you on the other side," he smiled.

The transplant worked beautifully. The color came back to his face. The irrepressible spark in his eye was brighter than it had been in years. He had his life back.

It didn't last for long. Things were still so experimental back in 1980. The doctors tried to adjust his anti-rejection medications. The kidney suffered and eventually failed. I would have given him the other one if they'd let me.

"I'll need you to take care of some things when I'm gone," he told me one night quite out of the blue.

"I'm not even discussing this with you Dad," I said angrily. "Don't you dare die on me, I can't handle it. I can't make it if you leave me."

I felt like a caged animal, scared and agitated. He had things he needed to say, but I wouldn't let him say them.

It was one of the only times I saw my father cry.

"You're my heart," he told me. "Please don't say that."

He fought like a warrior to stay alive. He had the last rites so many times it became our running joke.

"I'll go get Monsignor Danaher to give you the last rites again, Dad. That'll keep you alive for sure."

I never expected my father to die. He always came back. One night he called me from the hospital and asked me to stop by. "Is there anything you need, Daddy?" I asked.

"Just you baby, just you."

Those were the last words he ever spoke to me.

By the time I arrived at the hospital he was in a coma. I sat beside him and sang his favorite song, "Be my love." A beautiful piece sung by the late Mario Lanza. The song has a high "C" in it, and is considered very difficult to sing. Dad had always performed

85

it flawlessly.

He couldn't open his eyes as I sang to him, but tears streamed down his face.

"He can hear me Mom," I said.

I wanted to hope, but as the days went on the doctors told us there would be no comeback this time. We needed to say goodbye.

When we finally made the decision to take him off life support, Mom was the brave one. I couldn't stay.

"Go with God, Daddy. I'll see you on the other side," I said, stroking his hair through my tears.

I kissed him and I left my mother alone to watch him go.

The thought of dying didn't scare me quite as much after my dad died. My one shot at seeing him again. Having children changed that. When I was diagnosed with cancer I knew why he fought so hard to stay with me. I also knew how much pain I must have caused him by insisting I couldn't live with him gone.

SIX

Here Comes the Bald Bride

Donna's Journal
Home > Health
August 6, 2002

Hi folks!

Well... I got a sunburn on my head today! Took the kids to the beach to say goodbye to summer vacation... and instead said goodbye to my baseball cap on the crest of a big wave. I also scraped my knee. It was great! Think about it. When was the last time you scraped your knee. Made me feel downright young.

I get sort of sad at the idea of sending the kids back to school. Kind of sad and kind of ecstatic at the same time. Know what I mean? True to form my daughter is (mostly) looking forward to plunging ahead. She's organized down to the tip of her erasers. My son, meantime, keeps trying to convince me... I mean really convince me... that somehow a mistake was made... and that school is really another month away. I'm thinking of letting him have another month off. Yesterday he told me I look pretty... bald.

As I mentioned last week... I'm taking a few days off. So I'll see you next week.

Have a good one and God bless,
Donna

I was feeling good again. Another chemo break, but this time it was so I could enjoy the wedding.

"I was thinking Edith, it might be a nice touch if I could kiss the groom instead of throwing up on him," I smiled.

"Yes, yes, that could be arranged," she teased.

It felt strange though. All these delays because of my blood counts and here I was asking to put it off again.

"It's OK, Donna. Really," she said. "When you come back we will give you the necessary drugs to keep your blood counts up and we will go straight through to the end."

"And when exactly is the end Edith? You haven't really said."

I wasn't sure I wanted to hear the answer.

"Let's take a look at your marker when you get back, but I'm leaning toward a couple of additional chemotherapy treatments because of all the delays."

I knew all along this was a possibility, but I'd been trying not to think about it.

"I've always said you are a hateful woman," I said, raising what was left of my eyebrow in mock disgust.

"That, I am," she said, reaching out to hug me. "Have a beautiful wedding."

I purposely avoided talking about the wedding in my journal. It was one of those tough things about living in a fishbowl. I wanted it to be private. Not only for us, but for our families. We had both been through difficult very public divorces. We had hurt people we love, and I saw no need to cause more pain. The fishbowl thing is a double-edged sword. Of course the fact that people care about us is our livelihood. At that moment, all the caring was pulling me through one of the most difficult ordeals of my life. We can try to choose when to live in the fishbowl and when to draw the curtains, but it almost never works.

"Wedding Bells" was the caption on a local news magazine announcing our impending marriage. "Anchors to Marry" on another. Neither contacted us for the information. Both had the dates wrong, but it was out there.

For the record, Tim and I married August 9th.

"Good mornin' beautiful creature!" Marsha Coker beamed at me as she bounced down the stairs to the beach.

Marsha is a notary public. She is also one of our dearest friends. In Marsha's world there are no bad people. No bad days. No bad anything. To say she sees the world through rose colored glasses wouldn't be fair to her. She simply chooses to see the beauty in people. The rest would be a waste of her boundless energy. She and her husband Barclay have been married forever. They still behave like newlyweds. I have never seen two people who love life and each other more. Their love spills over to everyone lucky enough to be in their lives. When I was diagnosed for the second time, Marsha sent me a card every day for a week.

"Could the morning be any more spectacular?" she said clapping her hands.

Marsha would perform the ceremony with help from Barclay.

I was dressed in a white sarong, an aqua blue top and a white hat. Tim wore a Hawaiian style shirt with matching colors and white shorts. We had bought the clothes on our last trip to Costa Rica, a place that has become our home away from home. Neither one of us had tried them on before that morning.

"You nervous? You missed a few buttons there Timatao," I said.

"I didn't miss them, they weren't there," he grinned.

"Well don't feel bad, I put on my sarong and found it to be completely see-through. Luckily I'm so short I was able to double it and it still worked."

We laughed. The clothes didn't matter. We could have gotten married in pillow cases and we wouldn't have cared. It had been such a long road to get here, and although the cancer had thrown us a nasty curve it had only served to bring us closer.

Tim and I said our vows at sunrise, the "I dos" coming right on cue with the brilliant first rays of the disc on the horizon. At that moment, I was totally unaware that I was bald or that I even had cancer. I was just home.

We chose simple gold wedding bands. Simple, but not invisible. The reaction from viewers was immediate and gracious.

To: donnahicken@firstcoastnews.com
Subject: Fan

Hi Donna,
Glad to hear that you are doing well with your chemotherapy. I have been an avid viewer and fan of yours since moving to the beaches in 1994. Your courage, humor and vitality come through every night to your viewers when you do the broadcast.
I will continue to keep you in my prayers and wish you the best of luck with your treatment and your personal life. And on that note, I have one quick question and I hope you don't think it too personal. Did you and Mr. Deegan get married this past week and I missed the announcement on the broadcast??? Just curious, as I noticed you are now wearing a ring. Best of luck to both of you if you did, you make a GREAT COUPLE.
God Bless,
Betsy Slowey

To: Betsy
Subject: RE: Fan

Hi Betsy,
Thanks for the nice words I really appreciate you! And good eye! Yes... Tim and I got married last week. We didn't make an announcement... just preferred to keep it private... but I don't mind sharing one on one with nice folks like you. Thanks again for the support.
Donna

To: donnahicken@firstcoastnews.com
Subject: Congratulations

Hi Donna — Just a note to say congratulations on your wedding. I also wanted to say that the offer still stands if you need help with any design work for your foundation. I am happy to donate my time and talents to help you. Please let me know how I can help. I pray that you are feeling better and recovering from chemo. You are such an inspiration to so many.
Take care. Cynthia Montello

To: donnahicken@firstcoastnews.com
Subject: You and Tim

Thought I'd take a moment and tell you I heard some really great news yesterday. I wish you and Tim all the best in your new life together. I think it's great! Now how does a humble homicide investigator pummel this information out of someone??? hmmmmm :o)
God bless,
Rick

To: Rick
Subject: RE: You and Tim

Hey Rick!
Did you say humble homicide detective???
Isn't that a contradiction in terms?? OOOOOOOHHHHH... just kidding. It's great to hear from you. Thanks for the well wishes... I'm doing fine for a short bald girl. I hope all is well with you. Keep up the good detective work and the prayers! God bless you too and take care.
Donna

To: donnahicken@firstcoastnews.com
Subject: Don

Donna,
If my *Jacksonville Business Journal* is correct, I want to send my heartiest congratulations to you and Tim on your marriage.
Before Stereo 90 "bit the deck," Tim sent us a CD by Don Hazouri (I knew him!!) with a selection of his songs. He wanted us to play something for you to make you feel better. I am not certain the disc was played, but I did speak to Tim who was so eager to make your day better during a bad time. He was so passionate... I thought how caring one staffer was for another!
I played trumpet for the Jax Symphony and for a lot of Amelia Smith's opera productions. I knew Don Hazouri quite well, as a matter of fact, and didn't realize he was your dad. I suppose he's gone on to "the great opera aria in the sky" as I haven't heard from him in years.
I wish you and Tim greatest happiness, good health, prosperity, and sunset beaches. I really enjoy your excellence on First Coast News...it's the best. While you're anchoring, I am appreciating you and Tim, as well as the entire staff.
Thank you for being you. (You continue to be on the prayer list at St. John's Cathedral.)
All my best! Madge Bruner Hazen

To: MadgeHazen
Subject: RE: Congratulations!

Madge ... Thank you so much for taking the time to write and for so many nice words. My dad was my treasure. Yes he is gone... in body... I still listen to my CD and think of him every day. I remember well when Tim asked to

have the CD air. Unfortunately the quality of the tape it was taken from was just too rough. He had such a beautiful voice. I truly appreciate the congrats I hope you'll keep the prayers coming! Thanks so much. Your letter made my day. God bless.
Donna

There were dozens of e-mails like these. This one and a number of others actually came in weeks BEFORE we got married, people taking me to task for holding back on something that hadn't yet occurred.

To: donnahicken@firstcoastnews.com
Subject: Rejoice

Donna, first let me say that I am a huge fan of yours and have been for years. I admire the way you are handling your cancer, and think you are an inspiration to so many people out there. But I want to talk about something else. I have heard that you and Tim Deegan are married now. If this is true, I think this is great, but I notice neither of you wear rings and that you have not changed your name. I know there are a lot of people involved in your relationship with Tim (ex-spouses, children). But I still think you and Tim should be able to celebrate your commitment to each other and share it with your fans. I'm sure a lot of people would rejoice in knowing you two have started sharing your lives. I guess I'm just a romantic, but I think you and Tim should tell the world you are married and love each other very much. I just wanted to share these thoughts with you. So my advice to you and Tim: REJOICE, SHARE YOUR LOVE WITH THE PEOPLE THAT REALLY CARE FOR THE BOTH OF YOU.
Thanks for taking the time to read this e-mail.
Penny Keefe

To: PennyK
Subject: RE: Rejoice

Hi Penny
I saved your e-mail because I didn't want to tell anyone until after Tim and I were married. We've been engaged since October... but the wedding was not until last week! That's why we took a few days off. Anyway, didn't want you to think I was ignoring you... we just wanted a little privacy until after the ceremony. Thanks so much for your support. I truly appreciate it. The rings are simple but I hope you like them!
God bless,
Donna

All the well wishes, my new life with Tim, and of course that small matter of no chemo put me in an energetic mood. That Friday we decided to attempt the first Jaguars pre-season game. This was no small feat. Our seats were about a hundred miles up at the very top of Alltel Stadium. This was before the escalators were installed. Tim loved it because he could literally watch the weather up there, but for me, the climb was a marathon in itself. By the time I got to the top, I was ready for a nap. We could only stay for the first half because we had to get back to work. So about the time I recovered from the hike up, it was time to march back down. As we started our descent a woman sitting near us caught my attention.

"Get on that journal," she said.

I had skipped writing in it the previous week, and someone had actually missed it.

Donna's Journal

Hello!

Well I've been taken to task. I was leaving the Jaguars game Friday night and a very nice young woman scolded me. "You thought we wouldn't notice...but you didn't write in your journal this week!" She told me to get on the stick. So I hope she's reading.

I had a wonderful few days off. Thanks to all of you who took the time to write to make sure I was OK. You all are too good to me. My doc actually gave me a small reprieve on the chemo while I was off so I could enjoy myself and recharge.

Back to business this week. In fact... I know you've heard me complain about my blood counts and how they make my treatment drag on and on. Well, I'm about to start a new medicine that is supposed to keep the counts from dipping too low. If it works, I should be starting to make some serious headway in getting through this craziness. I sure hope so.

I think I have about four eyelashes left. I'm not kidding. It's getting more and more interesting trying to apply my mascara before the newscast. It's starting to look like I have one big eyelash on each side. Do you think I should just go for the fake ones? I haven't decided.

It really is wild going through all this in public. Some days I just wish they would remove all mirrors from the building. The truth is...I haven't looked at myself on tape since all this started. Sort of reminds me of when I was pregnant. The only way I was able to keep going on the air every day was to just not look. I'm really not feeling sorry for myself. Just sharing some practical survival stuff.

Time to get back to work. Thanks for reading. Sorry for the gap... I'll do my best to stay up to speed. Have a great week and God bless!

Donna

To: donnahicken@firstcoastnews.com
Subject: Jaguars

Donna,
Yes, I am reading! I'm the "young lady from the Jaguars game."

By the way, you look fantastic on television. I'll be honest, I didn't like your long wig at first, but it has grown on me. You cannot tell that your eyelashes have thinned. You have nothing to worry about. You are very beautiful.

Hang in there, you look great in person too!
God bless and I'll keep praying for you.
Catherine Corcoran

To: donnahicken@firstcoastnews.com
Subject: Looking Good

You are definitely "worrying" too much about how you look - you always look great, with or without eyelashes (I would never have noticed that - you are so tiny in person and tinier on TV that no-one can see you that close to notice eyelashes!). Your smile and personality more than make up for a few missing eyelashes!!!

We see a new wedding ring on your left hand - is maybe that the reason for the few days off to recuperate? I certainly hope so - life is too short to be alone, especially when dealing with illness.

Thanks for being so upbeat...I was just diagnosed with lupus today and I look at people like you who exude strength. Thanks for being you - and STOP WORRYING! With love, Patti Thompson

To: donnahicken@firstcoastnews.com
Subject: 'from Donna's Journal'

Hey Donna !
I can relate about the eyelashes or lack of! I remember running in the Race for the Cure in '99 at the beach when we were having the Red Tide. I had on my wig & a ball hat on top of that so my wig would stay on (it was windy) - which it didn't. I also was wearing my fake eyelashes (The cheap ones at Walgreens or Eckerds work pretty well. Just don't buy the really thick ones - they look really fake. Applying them at first takes a while too!). When I got to the luncheon they had afterward I looked in the mirror. What a sight I was. My eyelashes were half on half off, my wig on crooked. Well, you got the picture. Didn't matter - I was so proud of the fact I had beat my husband by two minutes & had had a dose of Taxol two days before.
I know how frustrating low counts can be when you just want to get through with the treatment. But, as you well know low counts mean the drugs are working!
Keep up the positive attitude!
Cynthia Launey

To: Cynthia
Subject: RE: 'from Donna's Journal'

Cynthia what a great story! I can't believe you actually wore all that stuff to run. Now that's brave!!! I'm afraid when I'm not here... I'm usually quite a sight. I have this red baseball cap that I wear just about everywhere. You are right though... beating your husband is as sweet as it gets!
Thanks for sharing... it was fun to picture you enjoying the day. God bless.
Donna

To: donnahicken@firstcoastnews.com
Subject: 'from Donna's Journal'

Donna,
Good luck with your chemo...My father-in-law, finally beat his prostate cancer after 2 years of radiation and chemo...He is now cancer free. Hopefully you will be soon...Your wonderful smile makes the evening news much more brighter. Hope to see you in section 432 again this year.
Also, congrats on your marriage to Tim. Hope you two enjoy a long life together.
Much happiness,
Bill O'Donnell

SEVEN

My Fishbowl Runneth Over

My fishbowl was overflowing. But not just with kindness and congratulations. Despite the fact that I told people in advance I was taking off for a while, I began hearing rumors about my health.

"Mom says the rumor of the week is that you have a brain tumor," Tim told me one morning shortly after our return.

"A brain tumor?"

"Yes, apparently you are gravely ill."

"Oh brother, I don't have it bad enough. Now people have to give me a brain tumor?"

This was no big surprise. I live, eat, sleep and breathe in public. I'm used to it. While I was gone, there was even a rumor I had died! I was once again in the thick of my chemotherapy, though, and I was in no mood.

"I'm sick of this craziness," I barked.

"People just care about you Donna," Tim said. "But there is a lot of that kind of talk out there. Maybe you could say something in your journal."

Donna's Journal

August 28, 2002

Hi folks!

Please forgive me while I rant for a few minutes. Time for a little heart to heart. I've always known that being on television meant that I would need to live life in more of a fishbowl than most folks. As I've alluded to in the past... some days in dealing with cancer... that's a bit of a bummer. But overall... with the amazing support I have received and family-type relationship I have developed with you... it's been way more a blessing than a burden.

That said... I suppose it's only natural that rumors can sometimes get started and once started they can become "fact" to a lot of people. Over the past several weeks... sometimes just when I take a day off... I hear that horrible stories about the state of my health are out there. Let me say... categorically and for the record... they are not true. One of the reasons I started the journal was to keep folks updated without talking about my silly self on the news regularly.

Those of you who have been faithful readers probably already know what's what. But for those who may have heard conflicting stories let me try again. My cancer reoccurred locally and was removed. After my surgery I received radiation therapy and am currently undergoing chemotherapy in hopes that it will not return.

Beyond that... I know of no lumps, bumps, bruises, tumors, measles, mumps, phlebitis, or hangnail! Please forgive the sensitivity. I am the first one to admit that there are no guarantees with cancer. I just want the "facts" to be the facts.

Thanks for putting up with me... I promise to be nice again someday! Have a great week and God bless.

Donna

This was as close to a temper tantrum as I could throw on-line. Of course I was preaching to the choir. The people saying this junk weren't the people following my journal, but I had to vent. I got more responses to this entry than almost any other.

To: Hicken, Donna
Subject: Donna's Journal

Dear Donna,
I just read your Aug. 28th Journal entry. I know you are frustrated - but I had to smile... I know first hand what you described in your journal about the rumors circulating regarding your condition! I can laugh now but 4 years ago when it happened to me it wasn't funny at all. I'm not a TV anchor but I am a pastor's wife, which places me in that wonderful fishbowl, too. In addition, I am a public school educator, which seemed to also open me up to the rumor mill. Where do they get all of these ideas?????

I remember someone being surprised to see me at a public function because they had heard that I was "confined to a wheelchair and not doing well at all." I continued to attend church, even playing the piano for worship services! So I don't know WHERE they got that one.

Then there was the person that called my school to inquire about the "music teacher position" because they had heard that the school had "lost" their music teacher to cancer. I was still teaching through my treatment!

Believe it or not, within the last 6 months someone called me to ask how I was doing because they heard my cancer was back and it had "spread all over." I could tell you many more - but you've already heard them!! :)
You might want to write the funniest ones down because you will be able to laugh at them farther down the road, I promise! But for now, hang in there and keep fighting. I will if you will!!
Sincerely,
Rhonda Gauger

PS: My eyelashes were the first thing to come back! :)
You look GREAT!

To: Rhonda
Subject: RE: Donna's Journal

Hi Rhonda!
Thanks so much for taking the time to share that with me. You really have made my day. I must have written and rewritten that journal entry ten times before I actually sent it. I know I shouldn't let it bug me. And what's more... I know I can never stop the rumors. I've dealt with them in some form or fashion for the entirety of my professional life (20 years!). Intellectually I know the best thing is to ignore them and go on. It's just when I think of my kids hearing this stuff it makes me a nut case. It's not fair to

them that mommy lives in a fishbowl. They are great and resilient and funny and wonderful. And they are dealing with this stuff so well. It's bad enough as it is... you know. Anyhow, there I go again!!! I really do take most all of it in stride. I will take your advice and start writing down the best. You are right... we could probably both write one heck of a book one day. And of course I will keep fighting... and getting strength from your fight as well. God has blessed me with so much. Sometimes I fail to fully appreciate it. Take care and again... thanks so much. Donna

To: donnahicken@firstcoastnews.com
Subject: 'from Donna's Journal'

Good Morning, Donna,
I have been watching you from the very beginning...and always have enjoyed your straight facing of the news... never inappropriately "chipper"... but serious when necessary. It has always "irked" me when someone pops from an upsetting story... to that chipper... "Now! On to something less upsetting." You have always given each topic its due respect.

Now, on to the Breast Cancer Issue.
I am an RN and have worked Oncology, ICU and Peds Oncology and ICU for many many years.
You are right... there are no guarantees in life.
I come from a family of eight children.
About the time I started Nursing School, my eldest sister was diagnosed with Breast Cancer, Adenocarcinoma, a sure death sentence. (She was 33 then... and her youngest child only three years old.)
Today, she is 74 and has four children, 5 grandchildren and even some great-grands.

About 10 years later, another sister was diagnosed with the same seriousness of diagnosis and life challenge... and resultant Radical Mastectomy, Chemo and Radiation. She is now 64 and is well tanned, tours and speaks (on TV as the "Angel Lady")... and just returned from Alaska. She has four children, 9 grandchildren and no great-grands as of yet.

Know that you are an inspiration to so many, and your courage (to continue to work) are so unselfishly admirable. Your work certainly operates within the framework of a certain amount of both "image" and even "vanity" and yet you are right there, good days and bad.
Know that every day I see you with an increasing respect and send good vibes and healing your way, as I am sure so many have done.

You are right... "ATTITUDE" is so much of the overall picture.
Take Care, and may you be blessed enough to see your precious babies reach their full potential and one day...lay sweet grandbabies in your arms.
Sincerely,
Judy Michaels, RN

To: donnahicken@firstcoastnews.com
Subject: RE: positive thoughts coming your way

I hope that you are doing well. Just wanted to say hello and that I have been thinking of you and praying for you. Whenever I think of you, I smile. I think it's because you exude such a glow of faith and a positive attitude - even when I know it's rough. It's one thing to go through this with your real family, but to share with your TV family like you do is just amazing- thank you. I've got to vent a little. We just got back from taking Jon to college. He loves it and I am so glad. I cried for two days, but I am better now.

My chemo put me into menopause so I am hanging in there with that. We just found out that we are positive for BRC1 after my two other sisters tested negative for it. So if we would have known I might not have had breast cancer at all. The genetics lab out west did the testing so I don't know what's up. That's a little discouraging. I leave Monday p.m. for my surgery, but I am ready to get it over with. Sorry to complain. I'll stop now!! "This too shall pass" is one of my favorite sayings. Also, I love "Don't worry about tomorrow, God is already there."

God Bless. Thank you for sharing in your journal. And thank you for putting up with rambling strangers like me.

With Warmest Regards,
Wendi Hollis

To: Hollis, Wendi
Subject: RE: positive thoughts coming your way

Hi Wendi!
You never need to apologize for venting to me. It gets very discouraging having to eat... sleep... and live this disease 24-7. What you see of me on the air is such a small part of my day. Believe me... I have my moments too! I'm praying your surgery goes well and I'm sending you lots of positive vibes!! It's always great to hear from you. Don't ever hesitate. Hang in there girl.
Your friend,
Donna

To: donnahicken@firstcoastnews.com
Subject: 'from Donna's Journal'

You are totally justified in your sensitivity to rumors — for some reason people thrive on this (they must not have a life of their own)! If it helps, we are glad to have you in that fishbowl to share your joys, your progress, etc. You are in our homes on a daily basis more than friends or family and you have all become like a family to us (otherwise we wouldn't let you in our dirty, messy houses so frequently). I'm sure I speak for the majority, that we just want you better, are glad you are doing well and pray that you will continue to do so. Keep your chin up — I went on an anti-gossip campaign in my own life about a year ago and lost two "friends" because of it, but am better off this way.

Thanks for sharing your wedding news with me — CONGRATS to you and Tim and may you have many, many happy years together. Keep those cool ties on your little surfer boy there!
Patti Thompson

To: donnahicken@firstcoastnews.com
Subject: FROM MARY MILLER

Hi Donna,
You and I seem to have the same attitude — beat it once, will do it again. I get the same "doom and gloom" look from some people in Fernandina. What we have is not nice, but we can beat it!!
Nuff said.
Like you, my cancer recurred near the breast, in one of four lymph nodes removed. I am really debating about radiation - I have heard of two people whose lungs got

burned and it took a long time for it to heal. One still has fluid on the lung, the other lived on oxygen for about a year. Just one quick question — how long did you do radiation? They are telling me every day, Monday thru Friday for seven weeks and mine is after, not before the chemo. Sometimes I get so confused, I feel the doctors just guess at what treatment is necessary!!

I am finished with chemo and have the whole month of September off. Of course, in the middle of this, our bank has been sold and we are having to go to training for new loan products and to learn a whole new computer system! Oh well, we will survive! Lots of love and best wishes to you.

Mary Miller

To: MaryMiller
Subject: RE: FROM MARY MILLER

Hi Mary,

I don't know your situation specifically... but from what I know about cancer and what makes effective treatment ... I would strongly urge you to do the radiation. They have special directed beams now that can avoid most of the lung tissue. Talk to your doc about that. It has become a pretty precise business. From what I am told... radiation is the best tool against localized cancer. We know it kills the cells that are hit. And we know where those cells are. Chemo is a search and destroy for anything that gets away... but there is no exact way to know how well it works. Beyond that Mary, it's no biggie. You may get a little sunburn towards the end of the six weeks. And yes... I had it every day for six and a half weeks. Obviously your body... your decision. But I'd give myself every possible shot to not get this stuff back. I know what you mean about docs making guesses. It is frustrating to turn

your life over to someone else... This though is a pretty tried and true treatment. It's what they have. Hopefully someday there will be something better.
God bless you girl... and thanks as always for the support.
Donna

Mary Miller was one of a handful of journal readers who had become a constant in my life. I knew I could count on her for a response. She was traveling this road with me literally.

Mary Miller's Story
by Amy Copeland

"Ya gotta take care of yourself; you can't count on doctors to do it for you. Believing in my doctor and not taking the bull by the horns like you should, I didn't do anything about it. And it kept growing."

For 63-year-old Amelia Island resident and mortgage loan officer Mary Miller, beating two bouts of breast cancer was all about taking responsibility for her health, then taking care of business.

An active career woman and grandmother, she wears her short golden blonde hair in a sporty style that seems perfect for her busy life. Her clear green eyes project self-assurance.

She's always been more independent than most people are. After a divorce at age 33, she spent the next ten years in Jacksonville, raising her son alone. "My family lived in Pennsylvania. I grew accustomed to taking care of myself."

Mary remarried in 1984. "I have a son, Jay, who's 36 years old and lives in Atlanta. Through my second marriage, Stan has three kids, Jeff, Clay, and Lori. Between the two of us, we've got eight grandchildren: Jordan, Jake, Ty, Kerry, Samantha, Ryan, Jacob, and Isaac."

Mary was first diagnosed with breast cancer in 1998. "It was a rather bad experience because almost a year before that I found a tiny lump, like a BB, next to my nipple."

She had told her family physician about the lump in January 1997. The doctor told her not to worry about it. By the time she went back in January of 1998 for her annual check-up the doctor suggested she have it looked at, but he never made an appointment for her at the hospital. "So I just finally called the hospital on my own and made the appointment to have the ultrasound."

The tests revealed the lump was cancerous, and would require a complete mastectomy. "If I had gone when it was just a BB, and demanded that it be taken out and biopsied, I probably would not have lost a breast. I probably would have just had a lumpectomy."

Her mastectomy was scheduled, and when she arrived at the hospital a woman at the check-in desk informed her, "You do know that Blue Cross Blue Shield considers this out-patient surgery?"

"Cut a boob off and throw 'em out! You are joking?"

The clerk told Mary that her physician, Dr. Robert Taylor, had already made the necessary phone calls to the insurance carrier and obtained approval for a two-night stay.

The practice of limiting hospital stays for mastectomies is common. "There is legislation going on now to change that, but it's true with all insurance companies; it's not just Blue Cross Blue Shield," Mary said.

"I didn't come to until probably three o'clock in the morning. I was out that whole time. How in the world could they throw you out of the hospital? A breast removal is out patient surgery? You have tubes draining from you! I mean, no wonder people have problems. It's awful."

Tests following her mastectomy showed the cancer had no lymph node involvement. Despite her doctor's recommendation for chemotherapy, Mary was hesitant. "I read, and I went on the internet, and something would not let me do chemo. I just couldn't."

Dr. Matthew Luke, her oncologist, called Mary at home and begged her to take the chemotherapy. If she did nothing, she had a

75% chance of non-recurrence and a 90% chance of non-recurrence if she went through chemotherapy.

The odds didn't suit her so she told him, "You're only saying 15% more! And then all the side effects of chemo? I'm going to pass."

"My family was upset. Everybody was upset with me," but she held her resolve and told them, "I'm sorry. I can't do it. I just can't do it."

She recovered without chemotherapy, and was free of cancer until May 2002, when she was diagnosed with breast cancer for the second time. "Dr. Taylor is the one who discovered it. He felt way under my arm, in my lymph node area – up in the pit and asked 'Have you felt that? You've got a lump there,' he said."

"I said, 'No.' I put my hand there and said, 'I still can't feel it.' I was just praying it would be scar tissue."

After having the lump removed, she learned the cancer was back. Unlike the first, this one was an estrogen-related cancer. "Then I went through all the tests, and they told me it was only in one lymph node."

Like Mary, her family was scared. Just as he had done the first time the cancer occurred, her husband, Stan went with her to the first visit to her oncologist. "He was always there if I needed him. The whole family was great. I had lots of prayers. There's nothing worse than when you get it the second time. That is really scary. You've been through it once, and it's been four years. You go for a check-up and you get that news. It's a lot more devastating than the first time around."

Breast cancer can defy the statistics. Mary had none of the usual things to watch out for, no family history of cancer. "There's no reason I should have breast cancer because all the answers were 'No' instead of 'Yes,' which really absolutely amazed me. Cancer hits anybody. With me everything was perfectly normal, as far as statistics go."

On Amelia Island the number of patients with recurring breast cancer was growing. Four of the six women going through chemotherapy with Mary at First Coast Oncology were recurring breast cancer patients. She thinks this should get more attention from both the medical community and the media. "Nobody even mentioned to me the first time I had cancer how many times it can come back. It's unreal. There are so many people I know, that if it's not them, it's their sister, it's their co-worker. It's too much!"

No place is exempt from cancer. "It has touched so many people on this island, it is absolutely unbelievable. First Coast Oncology opened offices up here probably just about the time I had my cancer the first time, and they're so busy now that they're expanding. The gal who does my blood work at Dr. Luke's office said some days she does eleven chemos."

Not only doctors' practices are growing but breast cancer support groups are too. "When I went to Bosom Buddies there were maybe ten women, and now friends say there are about thirty that are in the meeting, in this tiny community, in a four-year period."

After attending her local Bosom Buddies support group for three or four months in 1998, she volunteered to help other women. No one called her then, the need wasn't as great.

An opportunity to help another breast cancer patient did come in the summer of 2002. She saw First Coast News Anchor Donna Hicken announce the beginning of her second fight with breast cancer. They would both be going through chemotherapy and radiation treatments at the same time, and they both planned to work throughout the experience.

A news segment about Donna's on-line journal prompted Mary to get in touch with her. "Donna became my first e-mail buddy. I had never contacted a total stranger on the Internet. She must have had hundreds of people contacting her during her journal. The fact that she took the time to respond impressed me."

She felt more and more connected to Donna as they exchanged e-mails on drug side effects, hair loss, wigs, and low days. Donna's most supportive e-mails came when Mary was deciding whether to follow the treatment recommended by her doctors.

"Donna was willing to share her thoughts which were so similar to mine. Donna's type of support was great. Her positive attitude just reinforced mine."

They both underwent chemotherapy in the summer of 2002. Mary had a total of four sessions spaced once every other week. Almost a month went by with no hair loss. "And then one day, I'm in the shower, and all of a sudden my pubic hair is on my washcloth. Hey! Nobody told me about this! You don't think about your other body hair, but there's hair everywhere. Eyebrows, eyelashes, and everything.

"And I think the most upsetting, worse than the hair on your head, is when you lose your eyelashes and eyebrows. It makes you look washed out." She was relieved that they grew back faster than anything else.

Following the advice of a neighbor who had been through chemotherapy, Mary clipped off all her hair, once it began falling out. "Which is the best thing you can possibly do. There's nothing more depressing than having clumps falling out. It's awful. It makes you feel dirty, and you don't need that on top of everything else."

She was bald for most of the summer of 2002. Mary wore wigs to her job at the bank. "But the minute I got home, it was baseball caps. Going shopping, baseball caps. Wigs are very hot, especially in the summertime."

"When you don't have any hair to absorb perspiration, you just cannot imagine how much liquid comes out of your head as perspiration. It's unbelievable. I played golf through all this. I just had to take a towel along to wipe my head off," she grimaces, then adds, "and usually take two baseball caps along, because once the hat got wet, I got cold."

Not only did Mary stay physically active, she remained focused on her work at First South Bank. This was a definite help for her. "I have a high pressure job as a mortgage loan officer. I didn't have time to think about me, instead I thought about all of my customers."

"I've got a terrific boss in Wyndham Manning. He's wonderful.

His wife is a breast cancer survivor, so he knew exactly what I was going through."

About this time the bank was in the midst of a merger. Mary was to attend a training seminar in Tallahassee. She couldn't while undergoing radiation. Her treatments were every day. Instead, her boss had her go in September, the month between the chemotherapy and the radiation.

She never got sick from chemotherapy, but the radiation slowed her down a bit. "I missed one day of work because I got a little bit run down and caught a cold. That's it. One day of work."

She also had to cut back on her exercise routine during radiation. Since her treatment was at 8:30 a.m. every day for six weeks, it was too time consuming to walk every morning.

Stan supported Mary in her resolve to stay busy through her treatments. As always, her husband was there with her sharing their favorite activities. The one thing they gave up was sailing.

When they first met, they sailed often on their 34-foot boat, the *Sandpiper*. Once they even took a year off to live on their sailboat, cruising both the Florida Keys and Chesapeake Bay. "We sailed for many years and then both of us got into golfing and the *Sandpiper* just sat down at the yacht basin not being used."

They sold the *Sandpiper* in December 2002, at the same time she graduated from radiation treatments for the second invasion of breast cancer.

Stan and Mary try not to dwell on the threat that the cancer could return. "It's just something you put in the back of your mind and go on with your life. There is no way of telling when it's going to come back."

Worrying doesn't help, but her family's prayers did. "Pray to God. That works. That works wonders. I think it is so important to have a positive attitude and keep working. If you're going to sit around and say, 'Humph. Is it going to come back today?' you're running down your immune system. You've gotta go on with your life."

*　　*　　*

As did many of the journal readers, Mary gave me credit for courage I didn't really possess. What choice did I have but to persevere? What choice do any of us have? While the rumors about my health angered me, would I have been as angry if they weren't the source of secret fears?

The news from my doctor that week only served to make matters worse.

"Your marker is at 45 Donna," Edith reported. "It's not that high, but it's not normal."

"As if you need to tell me," I thought. I had the numbers memorized. I knew exactly what normal was and anything more than 38 wasn't good. I knew what was coming next. We had done this dance before.

"You know I don't like this test. It's unreliable. The numbers can be influenced by so many things. It's only a trend that would be significant. But it's what we have."

"I know Edith."

"I know you know, but I also know this scares you and it doesn't necessarily mean anything."

My confidence in that was zero.

"I'm assuming it does mean I'll be having those extra treatments."

"Yes, but I had decided to do those anyway. It's just the right thing to do.

I told you I want this gone for good. OK?"

My energy was flagging as I walked into work that day and then into "the office."

The office is the name I give to the ladies restroom. Whenever the girls need a talk, we head there. It was getting close to news time so I was just rushing in to do my make-up and balance "Jennifer" on my head. I opened the door to see my colleague of 14 years, Jeannie Blaylock.

"Hi J.B."

"Hi Donna."

"How was the wedding?" we both asked almost in unison.

We laughed.

Jeannie got married the day after I did. No, we didn't plan it. It just worked out that way. In fact, our lives always seem to do that. Jeannie and I were pregnant at the same time. Me at 5'1" the human bowling ball. Jeannie at 5'7", slender and graceful with a round center. We anchored together then and it was a hoot to see us. Because of my vertical challenges my chair has to be boosted to hoist me almost above the set. Thus my whole body up to my legs shows on camera. Not a good thing for a human bowling ball. Jeannie on the other hand, was only visible from mid-torso up. I could barely tell she was pregnant on the air and she had twins! Even then Jeannie would harass me about doing my breast self exams.

"Do you have to do that on the air?" I would ask her anxiously in the commercial break.

"Yes, Donna, I do, for the very reason that it bothers you to discuss it. Women have to talk about this stuff."

I griped about it, but I did it. In 1999 I found my own cancer, a small pea-sized lump. It saved my life, as it has saved many others.

Jeannie's Buddy Check program is now saving women all over the world. She is driven on this topic, for which I am extremely grateful.

Jeannie and I have shared more than joyful coincidences. We were both divorced at the same time as well. A draining and desperate time for each of us . Now, here we were again, sharing a life experience. Jeannie was radiant with her new found love. It was beautiful to witness.

"You look happy," I smiled. "I heard the wedding was picture perfect."

"It was absolutely wonderful. It was tough to come back to work."

"I know what you mean, but in my case apparently some people thought I took off because I had a brain tumor or some other fate worse than death."

"What?"

"People worry, and then when I'm not here the rumors start."

"Well, you've been in the business long enough to know you can't stop those. Don't let it get to you."

"Easier said than done," I sighed, and turned to apply mascara to my one remaining eyelash.

Amid all the e-mails that week was one from my friend Wendy Chioji. She is the Orlando news anchor who did her own on-line journal after finding out she too had breast cancer.

To: donnahicken@firstcoastnews.com
Subject: Hey!

hey, you... it's great to hear from you.. I'm sure you were a beautiful bride!!! can't wait to see pictures. :-)
you know, I think the tamoxifen is getting in the way of me getting totally back in to shape. I've been working hard at it, running intervals, hills, cycling, swimming, and I'm just not able to get ahead to where I was. it's frustrating, until you put it all in perspective. (but it's STILL frustrating.. I know you know what I mean). I am going to Toronto tomorrow for a long weekend with my mom.. she turned 60 in June.. a late birthday celebration... last year, I missed it by 8 months, so I'm getting better... Kelly and I have talked about coming up to visit you guys... my old co-anchor is there now, too, John O'Connor. he's lots of fun, if you ever run in to him, or feel like a fun lunch date.

how much more taxol do you have to go? does it keep your hair from growing in? did you do anything besides taxol this time around? here's something funny... remember the clinical trial I was on, the weekly lower dose of taxotere? I loved it... my hair grew back in during

treatment, and it didn't make me sick.... but the results of the research are back, and I guess 70-percent of people on my arm of the trial were sick as dogs... couldn't tolerate it. go figure.
WC

To: WendyChioji
Subject: RE: Hey!

Yes... that's what they are doing with me. Weekly. Because of my blood counts though... we've had to take lots of breaks. Now on constant neupogen and procrit... so we are starting to power through. No more breaks until the end. The answer is though... Edith hasn't decided yet how many doses since the break thing. Soooooooooo who knows. Just putting my head down and going... You know what I mean. I am also taking carbo-platin. It's the one that makes me sick... but you know... you expect that. It's the fatigue that is bumming me out. Makes me scared you know..that my body can't take it. I'll get there. I don't know about the hair... you know it does come back but I shave it off every time. Maybe I should let it go and see what happens. It all fell out at first...so I just assumed I should just keep shaving it. You have said a lot of nice things about your co-anchor... I may try to look him up at some point. Would be glad to include him in any plans when you guys come up. As far as the exercise goes... just keep reminding yourself it's temporary. I wish to God I could take tamoxifen. I used to dread the idea... but man... the success with that drug looks pretty exciting. So what...are you running a 5 minute mile instead of 4:40 :) Who cares... you are out there doing it... WAHOO!!! I do know it's frustrating though when you reach a certain level of fitness to have to start over. I feel weak as a

kitten right now. Just sooooooooooooooo ready for this stuff to be over!
OK. I'll stop.
Have a great trip with your mom.... tell Kelly hi..and when you come back... let's see if we can plan something.
Donna

Hearing from Wendy made me feel better. Like Jeannie, Wendy and I have so many connections it's spooky. She too had undergone a particularly long and grueling schedule of chemo and she was doing great.

It was exactly what I needed to hear.

Donna's Journal
Home > Health
September 2 , 2002

Hi friends!

I had a great e-mail "conversation" with a dear long time friend who just happens to do what I do. Yes we are both news anchors but the similarities don't end there. Not by a long shot. Get this. I'm giving you a little history here. We both entered the business about 20 years ago... both worked our way up from weekends to weeknight anchor positions at almost exactly the same time. Independently we both got into running... and triathlons and such. We had both just finished the Boston Marathon... in the shape of our lives... when we both found out we had breast cancer.

I was diagnosed before she was... so it was nice to be able to navigate with her the rough waters when you first find out. Now she's helping me. She's doing great... perfect check ups, thank God, since she finished her treatment.

I remember being really worried about telling her I had it again... because I didn't want her to be scared. Nobody ever wants to hear about somebody getting cancer again... because it makes them worry about their own situation. It's only natural.

But you know what? After the initial shock and billions of questions back and forth... there's just so much to be shared between women who have faced and continue to face this. She has been so great. Keeping in touch with me even when I've been too overwhelmed to respond. She's back to her marathons and triathlons... and her life... HER LIFE. Beyond the fact that I am thrilled to see her doing so beautifully... it gives me tremendous hope!

Sometimes in the midst of this disease you can forget your own best advice. This too shall pass. It is only temporary. I won't always feel like this. That's where the sorority of women who live with breast cancer every day are such a blessing.

I have told you before this has been a blessing in many ways. My friend is one of so many many examples I could give you. Life is good.

Have a good week and God bless.

Donna

EIGHT

Twisted Sister

Three in the morning. I lay in bed, wide awake, rolled into a fetal position. Then onto my back, my side, my stomach.

"You OK?" Tim whispered sleepily.

"Sorry, I didn't mean to wake you. I'm in so much pain. My bones ache so bad, it feels like someone is pushing on them from the inside out."

"What can I do?"

"Make it go away."

There was nothing to do for the pain. The medicine was doing its job well. I wasn't missing chemo anymore, but my bone marrow didn't appreciate the intrusion. It was cranking out white cells faster than the poison could kill them.

"What a perverse trick to play on my body," I thought.

"Why don't you take the day off, Donna? Just rest," Tim said.

"Because I don't want to take the day off. I can't rest anyway. My mind races flat out when I sit still and that's worse than the pain."

Tim knew this about me. Like everyone else, he just wanted to help.

Donna's Journal

Home > Health
September 9, 2002

Hello friends!

It's been such a busy week. Sorry I'm just getting to this week's journal entry.

I have good news on the chemo front. The drugs they've been giving me to keep my blood counts up are working and it looks like I will be able to stay on schedule for the duration. If the Lord wills... as my grandpa used to say... my last chemo should be around Halloween. Talk about trick or treat!

I've heard from a number of ladies who have taken the same drugs... and YES... they do make my bones ache! I'm told it's because the bone marrow has to work so hard. YES... I'm exhausted beyond description. YES... I feel like an alien has invaded my body. You are not alone!!! The most asked question I'm getting these days is "how the heck are you still working?" The answer is because it makes me feel better. It really does. When I sit still I get even more fatigued... so I don't sit still any more than I have to. Everyone is different. I totally understand that for some people the reverse is true. I'm certainly not saying what I'm doing would work for everyone... but it does for me.

Hey your girl is finally involved in the discussion boards as well. Only took me four months to figure it out... but hey... better late than never right? Truly, your words of encouragement and your own stories of survival are such an inspiration to me.

Gotta go...enjoy the rest of your week and God bless!

Donna

P.S. To those of you who complimented me on the fake eyelashes...I have to confess I decided against them. But thanks for trying to make me feel good anyway :)

The words flew off my fingertips. My resolve went with them. It's not that I didn't believe what I said. I just believed something different moment to moment. Some guy with a voodoo doll was poking pins in me and I was at his mercy.

Back at home, we were getting ready to move.

"Danielle, could you hand Mommy another box please, this one's full."

Moving didn't help my mood. All of my stuff, all of Tim's, had been crammed into every corner of my house since the wedding. Worse, we were moving to a condo, even less room for all my junk. We had started that fun weeding out process of keeping this and dumping that, when I came across a basket filled with letters.

"Mom, it's time to go!"

I put the basket back in the closet where I found it and took the kids to school. When I returned I had the house to myself. I retrieved the basket and looked inside. On the top was a laminated funeral notice.

> **Hazouri –** Rufus L. Hazouri, born August 30, 1912, and a lifelong resident of Jacksonville, died December 27th, at his home. He was the husband of the late Louise David Hazouri and the father of the late Donald R. Hazouri. He is survived by his son Larry Hazouri; his granddaughters, Donna Hicken, Michel Moses, Tara Hazouri and Michon Hazouri, his great grandchildren Danielle and Drew Hicken, Hill Moses, and Ryan and Amanda Hazouri, and numerous nieces and nephews. Mr. Hazouri was affiliated with the Roosevelt Grill on Ashley Street, Cash Building Material and Desert Rider Sandwich Shop on Bay Street where he was affectionately known as "Pop".

I forgot all about packing. My Uncle Larry and Aunt Donna had given me the letters after my grandfather passed away. He died two days after Christmas in 1999. I had given him a book, a pictorial history of Jacksonville, as a present on Christmas Eve. He marked his page, laid back his head to go to sleep and just kept sleeping. I was in the middle of my first round of chemo treatments then and never had the emotional strength to read all the beautiful cards of sympathy. Why I thought I did on this day, I have no idea. I opened the first letter.

January 11 - 2000

Dear Larry and Donna,
There is hardly any way we can express our sorrow at your great loss. He was like a big brother to me when I got back from the service and had no place to go, no home, no parents, no job, no clothes and nothing but a few bucks I had in my pocket. Your father and my sister Louise asked me to stay with them until I got my store started. I then lived in the back of the store. Once I tried to buy a dress shirt. No store had them for sale. Clothing was in short supply. I mentioned this to your father. He said go to Wittens. He might sell you one. I went to Wittens on Adams Street. He said he had none for sale. I said my brother in law said you might have shirts for sale. He asked me who was my brother in law. I said Rufus Hazouri. The manager came up and said "sell him a shirt." Well Larry - Speedy, Dana and I wish you and your family much health and happiness.

Uncle Vic

I folded the letter and put it away. Then I went to the top drawer of a chest in my room and pulled out a plastic storage bag. Inside was my grandfather's sweater. I had kept it just to savor his smell. A combination of cigars and garlic, and some cologne he always wore. I took a deep breath, soaking in all the memories that came with the scents, then put it on, wrapping him around me. I curled up in a chair and spent the rest of the morning reading about my grandfather with a box of tissues by my side.

"I'm scared, Grandpa," I said aloud.

I never told my grandfather I had cancer. His wife, my grandmother had died from the disease when I was four and I didn't want to frighten him. He never noticed the wig, which then, was much like my own short hair.

"It's all right doll," I could almost hear him say.

But at that moment, I didn't believe anything would ever be all right again.

I picked up the phone and dialed the newsroom.

"No way can I go in today," I thought.

I hung it back on the receiver before it ever rang, took a long, hot shower to soothe my bones and my spirit, and went to work.

At the station, I sat staring at my computer.

"I have nothing positive to say," I murmured to the screen. "Geez I'm pathetic. Who wants to read pathetic?"

I considered not writing in the journal at all that day. If I couldn't be upbeat, I didn't want to weigh people down with my own depression.

"But how honest is that?" I debated. "People will see right through you if you put on some phony act."

I could hear my father in my head.

"Be yourself, Donna. Some people will like you and others won't, but they'll know that what they see is what they get."

I proceeded to write what was my most intimate journal entry.

Donna's Journal
Home > Health
September 18, 2002

Hello folks!

Who would you like to hear from this week? The good twin or the evil twin? It's so strange. With this chemotherapy treatment I go through more moods in one day than a newborn does diapers. One minute I'm ready to take on the world and win... the next... I can't see the sun through the rain no matter what I try.

I was cleaning out my closet today... yes it's true. And I came across a bunch of cards from my grandfather's funeral. I remember it so well. I was in my first round of chemo back in 1999... I had just had a horrible allergic reaction to some medication... I got out of the hospital and just wanted to curl up in bed when I learned of his passing. I felt like someone had dropped a ten ton rock squarely on my chest. All those feelings came back today when I saw the cards. I sat in a chair in my living room and just sobbed. It made me realize how much I miss him... and I guess it made me feel vulnerable too. I almost didn't come to work today. Almost.

I constantly debate with myself how much to share with you in this journal entry. How much do you really want to know about how I'm dealing with this cancer treatment day to day. I'm beginning to get sick of myself... so I know some of you have to be sick of me.

That said... I'll tell you that I am facing this last month and a half of treatment with excitement and dread all at the same time. As I explained before...now that my blood counts are cooperating, I'm going straight through. In other words... between now and the end of October I will be having chemo about every week with the exception of one. To be honest, it's a little scary. So bear with me. I'm doing fine... I'm just a little bit crazy... but what else is new? I'll share what I can manage... and what I can't I'll just make a joke. You gotta laugh.

Have a great week folks and God bless.
Donna

My very personal offering received an equally personal response.

To: donnahicken@firstcoastnews.com
Subject: 'from Donna's Journal'

Hi Donna:
Just wanted to let you know my thoughts and prayers are with you as you go through this battle again. I remember all too well how hard it was at times to make it through the day. I remember it too well, in fact. When I was at the cancer treatment center Thursday...I met this elderly couple who sat next to me and we hit it off so well, and the lady had the same stage of breast cancer as me. She's having a tough time with Taxol.... I sailed through that one and she sailed through Adriamyacin/Cytoxan!!!!! Go figure. I was so sick off those drugs I wanted to go ahead and die. I look at photos of myself and can't believe I went through all that stuff...... even though I still get weekly treatments. I'm going in a couple weeks for my follow-up scans.... sure you know what I'm talking about and I'm getting nervous. Scared they'll find a new spot

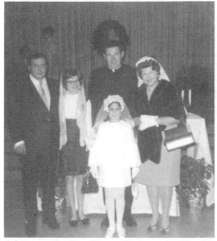

Above: L-R Don Hazouri (Dad), Elizabeth Hazouri (Mom), Monsignor Mortimer Danaher, Donna, Nancy Wright (Aunt Nancy) at Donna's First Communion, 1970.

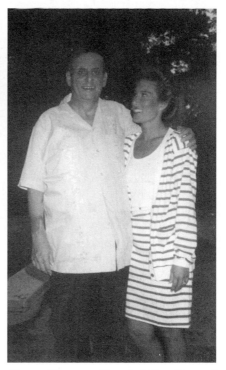

Above: Donna and her dad, Don Hazouri at the family home, Jacksonville 1989.

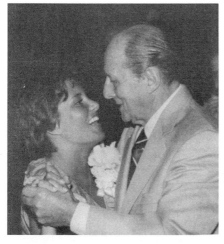

Above: Donna and her grandpa "Pop" cut the rug in 1983.

Right: Donna and her mother, Elizabeth Hazouri celebrating Elizabeth's "39th" birthday in New York.

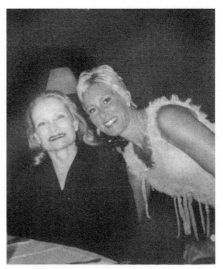

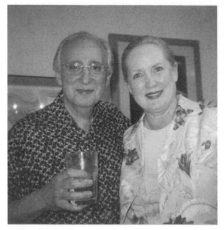

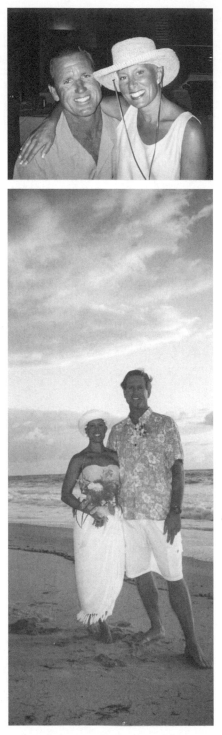

Above: Larry and Donna Hazouri (Uncle Larry and Aunt Donna), April 2003.

Upper right: Tim and Donna, August 2002. The Honeymoon.

Right: Donna and Tim at their wedding, August 9th, 2002.

Below: Barclay Coker, Marsha Coker.

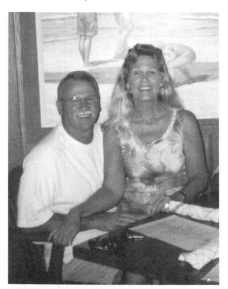

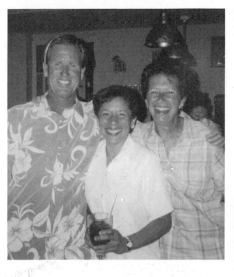

Left: Tim, Dr. Edith Perez, Susan Mehrlust at DHF Kickoff, June 2003.

Right: Carrie and Louis Wilson at their piece of paradise in Costa Rica, December 2002.

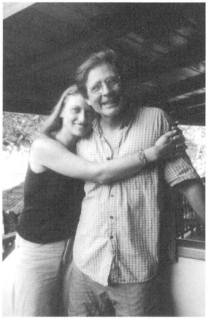

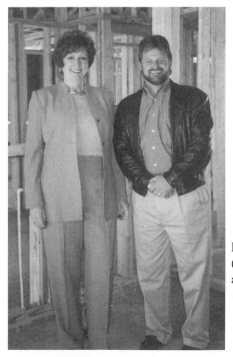

Left: Cynthia Montello, Paul Axtell (Classic American Homes) "Build Hope a Home" Fundraiser for DHF.

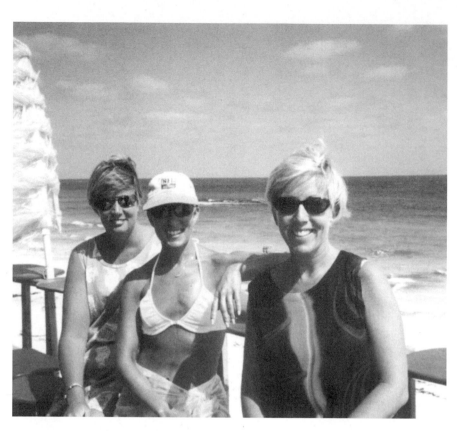

Above: L-R Celeste Beale, Donna, Julie Gillespie at Marsh Harbor, Bahamas for Post Chemo Get Away 2000.

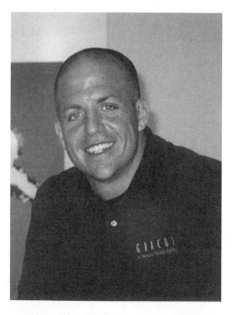

Right: Brett Chepenik, Donna's friend and Gracor Fitness Trainer.

Right: Donna and Nancy Bauer - River Run Finish March 2000. *(Photo courtesy Stuart Tannehill, The Florida Times-Union)*

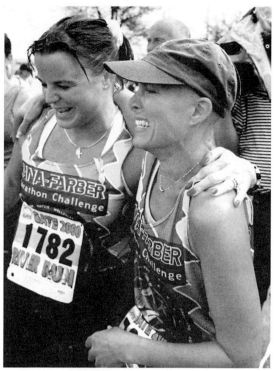

Right: Donna and Andrea Cole after Donna finished the Boston Marathon April 19, 1999.

Below: Jon Frankel in Hawaii at the Ironman Competition.

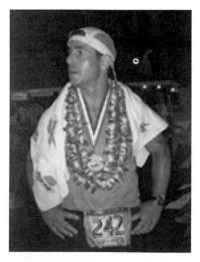

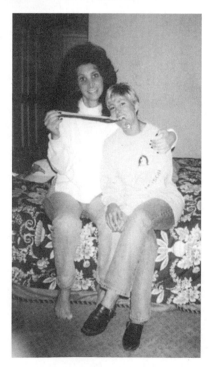

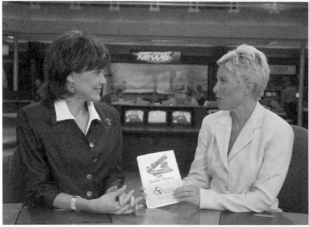

Left: Donna and her co-anchor Jeannie Blaylock talking up self breast exams with Buddy Check 12.

Right: My colleagues. L-R Mark Collins, Helen Garrard, Mike McCormick at DHF Kickoff, June 2003.

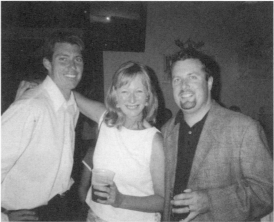

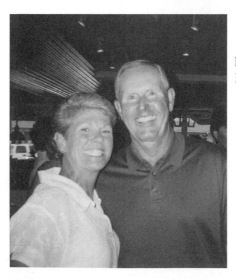

Left: Judy and Tom Coughlin at DHF Kickoff, June 2003.

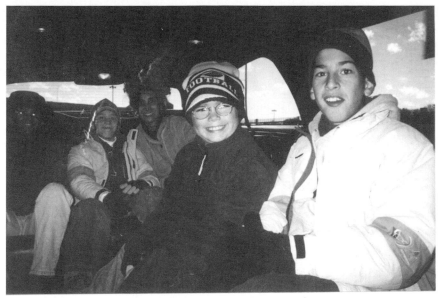

Above: "The Crew" in the limo in NYC. L-R Nancy Saalfield, Michael Gilbert, Andrea Cole, Drew Hicken, Christopher Gilbert.

Below: Donna and daughter Danielle ice skate in New York, November 2002.

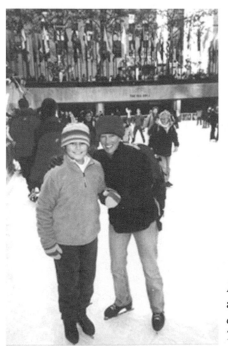

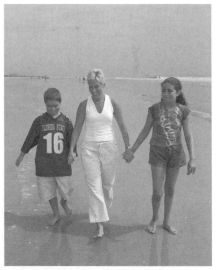

Above: Drew, Donna, and Danielle take a walk along Jacksonville Beach. *(Photo courtesy Reggie Jarrett, The Florida Times-Union)*

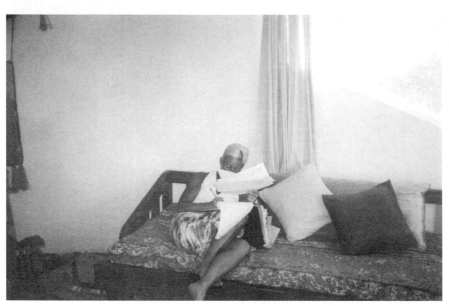

The Author at work.

Tim surfing.

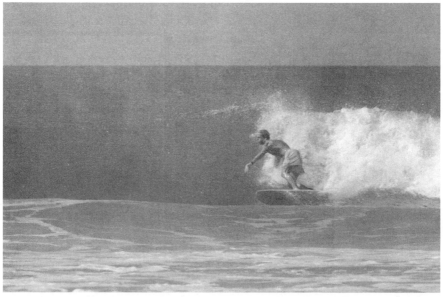

but at the same time, I want them to catch it as early as possible. Too many ups and downs, huh? Feel like I could conquer the world one day and feel like crawling under a rock the next. I know how you feel, but rest assured you are cared for by many people. Heck, no one knows me...... but I'm happy that you can tell your story and get the word out about breast cancer. It's so very important for all women to know what this cancer is all about. For some reason..... I run into women all the time that never ever examine themselves. their reason? Scared they'll find something. I go crazy when they say stuff like that. I have even spoken to nurses that don't do self exams!!!!!!!!! Can you believe that? Even my 4 sisters don't do self exams..... all because they're afraid they'll discover something. I'm amazed. I still spread the word to anyone that'll listen, and you know what?.... women I've spoken to about breast cancer have been very interested in everything I've said. I am so glad I can teach others about this disease. That's why you should be proud of yourself, too. You're doing a good thing by sharing your experiences and giving women out there a glimpse into "our" world. Take care, and my prayers are with you.
Tanya Wilcox

P.S. Thanks for responding to my post on the message board

To: donnahicken@firstcoastnews.com
Subject: 'from Donna's Journal'

I was reading your journal entries and read the one about coming across reminders of your grandfather, otherwise known as "Pop" to those of us who knew him. There's not a day that goes by if I go in Desert Rider that I don't

feel his presence there. I used to be in the bldg. right next door to him but moved across the street this past June so I don't go in there as often. but when I do I can see him waiting on people, driving those girls crazy in there. But they all loved him, just as his customers did. Rufus is feeding everyone in Heaven real well!! Just wanted to tell you that.
Cathy Hazouri-Weyand

To: donnahicken@firstcoastnews.com
Subject: 'from Donna's Journal'

Hi Donna – I just read your journal and want to say how brave I think you are. You are going through a lot, you cannot help but go up and down in how you deal with it. I went to counseling after our 3 month old son Blake died in 1990 and learned that journals were very helpful to clear your mind and kind of get it all out. (Plus we all want to know how you are so that we can be there for you!) Often when I come across cards or something of Blake's I still get teary, but then I'll find a tiny feather INSIDE my house on Mother's day! Or I'll just know he's helping me through my latest struggle. I think of my own grandfather so often and think he also picks me up when I am overwhelmed. Tears are cleansing and necessary I think. So just don't be too hard on yourself and know my prayers are with you as you get through these next few weeks. Take care and thanks for sharing with all of us.
Love, Nancy Buckler (San Jose Catholic)

P.S. Samantha (my 8 year old) was thrilled when you sent a note to your "fellow Trojan" last time we e-mailed. She keeps you in her prayers nightly too. Hang in there!

To: donnahicken@firstcoastnews.com
Subject: Hello again...

Me again, Patti... just wanted to let you know you can't share enough, as far as I am concerned... when we hear your downs that just tells us out here in TV land that you are human, just like everybody else. My Mom is taking chemo for lung cancer, as I said before, and she says to tell you she is with you 100% and to please tell you that (she doesn't have or want a computer). She went to Mayo one day a while back for chemo and saw you with Tim with beach gear and came home so excited - she was so thrilled to see you both in person! She couldn't even remember what Dr. Tan had told her about herself! Y'all just have a way with your fans!

Turn those grandfather tears around girl, and think about the wonderful memories you have of him. I know you do - remember each tear was an angel crying with you, telling you how much your grandfather is with you everyday and sending his healing prayers down to you. I was very close to my grandmother and she comes to "visit" - she smells like toast and has appeared to me in Dillards, Publix as well as all over my house. I am not crazy!!! (I see what you mean about sharing too much information) - I love to have her around. Your grandfather just appeared then to help you clean out your emotional closet - good healing.

Good girl with the other closet - I have to do that too. In the same category with the mud roll and bug eating. I have a dress that I made in the 70's, a size 8 (when a size 8 was like a size 2 now - it would probably fit you) that won't fit my right arm now - why do I still have it? It must have served a purpose somewhere along the line, along with the bell bottoms...

Anyhow, you can never share too much with us - we are with you through thick and thin and you are just letting us know that you are human like everyone else. I don't think you can really grasp how many people out here are pulling for you and really care, not because you are a TV personality, but because we just genuinely like you and your strength, your feisty, your humor - you are just a good gal and we all want to keep you around.

So pack up those woes and toss 'em out with the closet rejects, keep us posted, and if you feel a crying jag coming on let us know, and we'll all cry with you.

Will let you get to work now and I have to get back to that peach quilt I'm making... are you a peach person? You look like you could be...
God bless and keep you,
Patti Thompson

To: donnahicken@firstcoastnews.com
Subject: 'from Donna's Journal'

Well I will pray for you "twisted sister," my Sign class at FCCJ, is following your Journal, and I honestly wouldn't have ever stopped to read it if it weren't for my teacher. I am glad that I did though. "Eye of the Tiger." I will continue to follow your Journal now and I know that you can make it.
Tori Powers

To: 'donnahicken@firstcoastnews.com'
Subject: 'from Donna's Journal'

I just read your September 18th journal. Thank you for being honest and real. I know you are helping many who are also going through various treatments. When my father went through radiation and chemo several years ago, it was hard for both of my parents. They had no idea what to expect. My father's cancer was not caught in time and we lost him seven months to the day after the diagnosis.

I hope you will turn your journal into a book so you can share with those fighting the cancer monster. Let them know it is okay to have bad days. And it is okay to have good days. But most of all to show them that there is VICTORY. Be blessed!
Glenda Dean

To: donnahicken@firstcoastnews.com
Subject: 'from Donna's Journal'

We don't get tired of you. We miss you when you're not on the news; we've been there, so to say. So we wish you all the best. We, like so many others, hope you keep the cool and keep fighting. We love you. We are praying for you.
Bob & Linda Lewis (Melrose, FL)

To: donnahicken@firstcoastnews.com
Subject: 'from Donna's Journal'

Hi Donna,
I just wanted to say hello to the bravest, most beautiful girl on the air!! By the way, Jennifer looks great!! I finally

ditched Edna. I have a little boy hair now, so I decided the heck with it! Well, we had an encouraging and positive "pow-wow" at Dana-Farber a couple of weeks ago. They are still trying to figure out what is going on with us!! I feel better and better everyday- but that fourth and last chemo just about knocked me out!! My next big thing I think I told you is my surgery On Sept. 11th. I'm trying to decide what size to become- I told my husband sorry no Pamela Anderson!! We are taking our oldest Jon to college on the 29th- I will miss him terribly, but I am so excited for him. Our daughter Jordan will turn 13 on Sept 12th(we feel so terrible missing her birthday- we are going to make it up to her somehow!!).

Thank you for your journal. It is so nice to know how you are doing. As always the prayers and thoughts are coming your way. They come to you on special little angel wings. Oh, by the way, try to check out the September *Reader's Digest* when you get a chance. There is a story in there called "Another Chance to Live" -I think. It features my oncologist-Eric Winer and my surgeon-Dirk Iglehart. They are wonderful, caring doctors. Actually, I know there are wonderful doctors in Jacksonville, but my sister worked at Duke with Dr. Winer when we lived in N.C. and so we just stayed connected to him through all three of us girls as we've gone through our cancer. God Bless You!! I hope school is going well for the kids!

With Warmest Regards,

Wendi Hollis

To: Hollis, Wendi
Subject: 'from Donna's Journal'

Hi Wendi... I just feel compelled to tell you that your letters always make me smile. You seem to truly love life and it shines from you like diamonds. Thanks for sharing!!

Does your husband get a say in the cup size sweepstakes?
I'm looking forward to hearing what you decided. Keep
smiling girl... you are a real spirit lifter. God bless.
Donna

Wendi Hollis was another all-the-time e-mailer. A survivor.
She was a vivid writer, I could always see the scenes she painted
for me. Over the months, she shared her family's very personal
pain. Yet, it always seemed that lifting me from mine was her top
priority.

Wendi Hollis' Story
By Katrina Mims-Cook

"I heard a gentleman say one time that we're here to love each
other and serve each other. I try to live by that. I realize that life
really is too short," Wendi Hollis says. Her voice is soft like the
light breeze blowing through the moss lined trees that column the
covered seating area behind Bolles School.

Wendi, a 41 year-old wife and mother of two, was diagnosed
with early stage breast cancer in November 2001. She is the oldest
of five sisters and the third to be diagnosed with the disease. Her
sisters were diagnosed, Cindy in 1994 and Kristy in 1999.

"I was reading one night. I had an itch and my fingers brushed
a hard lump. It was at the very edge of my right breast," Wendi
Hollis says, tapping her finger on a spot near the middle of her
chest. "I shook my husband awake and said, 'Chuck I found a
lump.' We just looked at each other."

After a core biopsy confirmed that the lump was a small invasive
ductile carcinoma, Wendi contacted Dr. Eric Winer at the Dana-
Farber Cancer Institute in Boston. Dr. Winer had worked with
Wendi's sister Kristy during her nurses training at Duke University
and he treated both Cindy and Kristy for their breast cancers.

Telling her children about the biopsy results was one of the
most difficult things she had to do. Her son, Jonathan was a senior

in high school, a baseball pitcher for Bolles and was being recruited by a number of colleges and Ivy League schools. Her daughter Jordan, 12, was just starting sixth grade at Bolles. "When someone in your family is diagnosed with a disease like cancer, it's like everyone in the family has received the diagnosis. It changes everything," Wendi said.

She told Jon first, "We were watching a Notre Dame football game in the family room. Chuck and I had planned to talk to him together, but it just felt like the right time. I will never forget the look on his face when I told him about my cancer. The first thing he did was hug me. He said, 'It's going to be okay and we'll do whatever we have to do.'"

Her voice catches when she recalls telling her twelve year old daughter. "I'd sit on her bed and stroke her hair while she was sleeping and pray for the right words to tell her. I'd go to her doorway and think this is the child who loves the Disney Channel, who loves to play the Nancy Drew computer games with me. How do I do this to her?"

Wendi feels that seeing her two sisters recover so well from their breast cancers helped both Jon and Jordan cope with the news of her diagnosis and the traveling involved with her treatment.

In November, Wendi and Chuck met with Dr. Winer in Boston. He outlined a course of treatment for her that would include four cycles of Adriamycin Cytoxin once every three weeks. "I told Dr. Winer that I didn't have time for this and I asked him if I could delay the treatment until Jon graduated from high school. He said, 'Do you want to see him graduate from college?'"

Wendi and Chuck returned to Dana-Farber on December 20, 2001 for her lumpectomy. "Before we left, Jon gave me his St. Christopher medal. Jordan gave me love notes and her rosary. Mom pinned a medal on my shirt over the tumor and my sister Kristy gave me a wooden cross. Other family members and friends called and made me laugh and sent loving prayers. My father made all the travel arrangements so we didn't have to worry."

The stark reality of what she was about to undergo hit Wendi the night before her surgery during the taxi ride from Boston's

Logan International Airport. "We were listening to a news-talk station in the car when a voice comes on the radio and says, 'An estimated 40,000 women will die of breast cancer this year.' I just burst into tears. I mean, I had been fine, but it was so in my face that I started crying."

Wendi had a sentinel node biopsy before the surgery, a procedure that she says was not available for either one of her sisters. "There are things that have dramatically changed in treatment and procedures from when Cindy was first diagnosed in 1994. There are things that were available to me that weren't even available to Kristy just four or five years ago."

The sentinel node biopsy shortened her recovery time and left Wendi with little pain afterward. She was able to fly back to Jacksonville without pain medication just hours after the surgery.

A few weeks after her second chemotherapy treatment, Wendi began losing her hair.

"It was on a Saturday afternoon. My head was itching and my hair was coming out in clumps. Jordan said, 'Mommy just let me shave it. It'll make you feel better.' We put the kitchen chair in front of the television and while we were watching the Disney channel, my daughter shaved my head."

The hair loss was greater than she anticipated. "That was the one thing I was most mortified about. I was trying to keep the life routine normal and by losing your hair, obviously people know something's wrong. But it was such a relief when it was gone."

Wendi's son, a senior in high school, had his head shaved that same day to show his support. "My family would say, 'Oh you're beautiful without hair.' Here I feel like a Martian and they're saying, 'Oh honey, you have a beautiful head,'" she recalls, laughing.

Jet engines thunder overhead interrupting her reverie. Military planes come into view and her eyes follow their path. She shifts in the seat, adjusting her navy blue walking suit. Her soft, hazel-green gaze becomes intent.

"If there seems to be a lack of tears and hysterics it's not because there was a lack of emotion. There was very deep emotion, but also very deep faith in the Lord."

Her trust in God, along with her husband's strength and stability got Wendi through the difficult times. "Chuck was extremely calm and really my rock. I can remember sitting on the bathroom floor so sick from chemo that I couldn't move. He'd sit there with me wiping my tears. His job was extremely supportive, they gave him time off whenever he needed to be with me. We have good insurance through them, that was a huge relief."

Her family was equally supportive. "My mother and sisters would keep a vigil by my bedside bringing me Sprite, Jell-o, popsicles and crackers. My father would run errands and pick up whatever we needed."

Wendi's nose wrinkles slightly as she recalls one of the not-so-good times. "That's not to say we don't have our moments of 'this totally sucks', but they're very rare. An associate of Dr. Winer's in St. Augustine did my chemotherapy treatments. I felt awful in between the treatments. I felt like a Zamboni machine, that cleans ice hockey rinks, was running over my body."

Taking charge of her health care, Wendi made the decision to have both breasts removed. "Before my surgery I said, 'Honey, are you going to mind if I don't have breasts?' And he said, 'Honey, I just want you here.' Chuck is such an awesome husband. He would make me feel attractive wearing a bag."

She had a double mastectomy on September 11, 2002. When she came out of recovery, Chuck broke the news to her that the doctors had found another small tumor, this time in her left breast.

"Originally it had been in my right breast. This was totally out of the blue. Mind you, before any of this, I never felt sick. That's what's so deceiving. I never felt sick a day before my diagnosis. I got yearly mammograms and I had the Buddy Check 12 chart hanging in my shower."

Wendi had to undergo chemotherapy after the double mastectomy, this time twelve weeks of Taxol. "My hair had just started to grow back. It was about three inches long," she says, tucking a contrary strand of shoulder length chestnut brown hair behind her ear.

With a family history of breast and ovarian cancer, Wendi opted to have a prophylactic hysterectomy after completing the Taxol treatments. Just this past summer she underwent breast reconstruction surgery.

Wendi feels that angels have been camped around her since the day she was diagnosed; guiding and encouraging her. Head tilted slightly and with tenderness in her voice, she tells about the kindness of her friends, family and the Bolles School community.

"During my chemotherapy treatments, Jon's baseball team was traveling around Florida playing in the regional tournament and then the state tournament. Going to watch those boys play was the best medicine for me. Cheering them on helped keep my mind off my cancer. That was truly the best of times and the worst of times for us."

Since being diagnosed with breast cancer in 2001, Wendi has come to rely on the support of the cancer survivors in her family and the friends she has grown close to along the way. Wendi's friend, Rae Stopyra, arranged for huge boxes of casseroles, breads, salads and desserts to be delivered from the school. People prayed at their churches. Flowers cards and gifts came. "The community was wonderful to my whole family."

Richard Lewis is a special gentleman she met at a Bolles baseball game. He has Leukemia and is now battling cancer. "Richard would call and encourage me, but he would never talk about himself or complain. As he was leaving a game one night he turned to me and said, 'I want to tell you one thing that I don't want you to ever forget. Never give up.'"

Wendi believes God puts special angels like Richard Lewis and Donna Hicken on the earth to help us. "Donna is like the leader angel and I am so blessed that God put her in my path."

One night after seeing Donna on TV, telling the First Coast viewers that her cancer had come back, Wendi e-mailed Donna. She had just been diagnosed with breast cancer, so the announcement had a great impact on her. "I felt like she was talking to me. She was saying that her doctors had been annoyingly diligent and had found more breast cancer and they were going to do the hair experiment again. I just cried for her."

Wendi was encouraged by Donna's strength and positive attitude. "She was that person that I could look to every night for inspiration. I would think if she can be on the air doing the news, then I can get up off the couch!"

She started reading Donna's weekly journal. "She was refreshingly honest and she wrote about the most hysterical things that mothers go through. She also wrote about the struggles of others. I would read the journal and laugh, cry and be thankful that she was there for me. This courageous woman was reaching out to us in the midst of her own fight."

*   *   *

The words were air for me that week. They literally kept me breathing.

I was at mile 18 of my marathon. The wall. It's when even the strongest runners can convince themselves they are done. The body is depleted of all it's reserves. The finish seems just out of reach. The thighs are burning. The lungs heaving. The runner's legs are turning on pure will.

"When you think your legs are giving out, visualize yourself breathing oxygen into the muscles," Brett would tell me.

People gave me that oxygen.

Chemo took it away.

"Your face is starting to look a little flushed, Donna, you OK?" Tim asked.

I shook my head.

"Want me to get the nurse?"

I nodded.

Suddenly I couldn't breathe. Someone had tightened a noose around my neck and I was gasping. Trying to gasp. It was like trying to breath through a cocktail straw. My face was swelling. Someone was pressing on my eyeballs from inside my skull.

My chemo nurse Jim came flying into the room. Slapped oxygen on my face and something into my IV.

138

Tim looked at me, helpless. I stared back like a deer in the headlights.

"Breathe the oxygen Donna, slowly. Just breathe. You're OK." Jim had his hand on my shoulder.

The noose was loosening. I could feel it sliding off my neck. The pressure in my head ebbed away. I took a long satisfying drag on the oxygen. My breathing returned to normal.

"What just happened?" Tim was still stunned.

"Allergic reaction," Jim said.

This had happened to me once before, only much worse. It was right after my first diagnosis. My very first round of chemo. Edith was excited about a new drug called docetaxel. I was part of a study that allowed me to take it. The nurse had put no more than a teaspoonful into my veins and my body went into shock. I thought I might die that day.

The memory of that made this episode even scarier. It never got as bad, but the fear was there.

"We are going to have to take you off the carboplatin Donna," Edith told me the next day.

"But why? We were able to override the reaction and continue, and will that make the chemo less effective?"

I was upset. I didn't want to change drugs in the last month of my chemo. Edith was convinced the combination we were using was the perfect one-two punch to knock out the cancer for good.

"We have no choice Donna. This has happened before and women have died. We were fortunate to control the reaction this time. Next time we might not be so lucky. We simply have to hope that the drug has done its job. You can continue with the paclitaxel."

The news was sobering. Unavoidable. The one positive was that the drug I was giving up was the one that made me so nauseated. The paclitaxel was much easier to tolerate.

"Let's focus on that," Tim said as I filled him in at home.

"Let's focus on that nasty garage," I replied.

We only had a few more days before our move and the garage was far and away the biggest mess.

"I'll get going out there," he said. "Why don't you tackle that hall closet?"

That sounded good to me. When I opened the door it didn't look like too much work. Closets are deceiving that way. You don't realize you are actually getting sucked into a black hole. Every time I thought I had come to the end, there was one more shoe box stuffed with something. Mostly things the kids had made. I would head toward the "dump" pile and then always turn back. I've never been able to throw memories away. It was inspiration for my next journal entry.

Donna's Journal
Home > Health
September 24, 2002

Hello friends!
I couldn't possibly begin to thank you for all the words of support I've received this last week. Support almost doesn't seem strong enough. I feel as if I have my own flock of guardian angels hovering over me all the time and keeping me looking up. You are just the best.

It's been a wild week. I'm in the middle of moving (that's the ONLY reason I was cleaning my closet last week :) and it's just amazing to me how much stuff one can collect. I remember starting out with the firm purpose of amendment that I was only going to have one junk drawer...just one! I think at last count I had about 12!!! I admit it, I am in fact the original pack rat. I can't throw anything away. If my daughter put her handprint on a picture in pre-k... or my son made a paper pilgrim... I've got to keep it. Problem is... they did that every week. I can't help it... I just can't toss that stuff. And I've raised them to be just the same. It seems a harmless enough habit...until you try to box it all up and move it somewhere else. I get these big wet eyes looking back at me...

mommy I KNOW I haven't played with that in three years... but I really need it. What are you going to do?

I got the greatest e-mail from a nice woman who shared her grandma's advice after a wild day with the kids. "Oh honey...the first hundred years are the worst". I think that's such a hoot. And certainly true. After that it's all cake.

Have a great week and God bless.
Donna

The week that followed was exhausting and exhilarating. We finally closed on our new place, loaded up our lives, and moved them to the ocean. I have always dreamed of living here. The ocean is peace to me. It has more moods than a chemo patient, but it's constant at the same time. I can have the worst possible day, and just stepping out onto the balcony to see it, smell it, taste it, can calm me more surely than any drug. I took our moving day off to get things organized. Tim came home at dinner time.

"Is it still there?" he asked making anxious strides to the balcony.

"Yes, it's still there," I smiled.

The question has become a daily ritual, and sure enough, the ocean never disappoints us.

Donna's Journal
Home > Health
October 1 , 2002

Greetings!

Well I survived the move and am now trying to maneuver my way around a mountain of boxes. I keep reminding myself of my mantra these days...just take 'em one at a time.

Speaking of which... my countdown officially begins today. Four weeks from today it's D-O-N-E! I will have my second...and Lord willing... final "no-mo chemo" celebration. The last time I had a huge party, which just happened to fall on tax day (April 15th).

As I think back it was such a different experience the first time I was diagnosed. I don't think I ever seriously considered facing this again. I had a small tumor, no positive lymph nodes and no real history of breast cancer in my family. I considered the surgery and subsequent chemo and radiation a slam dunk. What is the saying? Life is what happens while you're making plans. It's true. This time... even though my cancer is still considered "local"... I'd be lying if I told you I had no doubts about whether this will ever return.

I was talking with my doctor about that the other day. Should I prepare myself for the possibility that this may come back... or do I tell myself... like last time... I'm done... really done? The latter... she said. You go on with your life... and you don't worry about what ifs. Otherwise... you forget to live. I think that's great advice. I'm going to do my best to follow it. I'll unpack what the days hold one at a time... just like the boxes.

Have a great week and God bless.

Donna

NINE

My Miracle

Funny thing about a marathon. You'd think after running 25 miles the last 1.2 would be a celebration. Pure elation at having nearly completed such a long and grueling task. But at least for me, those last steps seem like the elusive search for the holy grail.

"I should be there by now. Come ON."

A half a year of my life was gone. I was in the homestretch of chemotherapy. Only two treatments left. But what then? The anticipation of the finish was there, but with cancer, so was the fear.

While I was marking time, my friend Jon was counting down to his Ironman.

I was living vicariously through him. Wishing my body was capable of doing something so amazing. At that point, one mile would have been a victory for me. Heck, one tenth of a mile.

I had sent Jon a T-shirt early in his training that showed all the triathlon events with the caption "multi-tasking." Just before he took off for the event, I left him a message telling him my chemo was winding down and wishing him luck.

"Leave it on the road," I said. "Give it all you've got and don't hold anything back." I received this e-mail back from Hawaii.

143

To: donnahicken@firstcoastnews.com
Subject: Leave it on the road

I'm glad you are nearing the end.
I'm sure you've been a champ about it
I'm so sorry you have to go through this again.
I don't think I'll have any choice but to leave it on the road – literally.
Although that is one of my goals: no cramping, no throwing up..
You can track on IRONMANLIVE.COM – my number is 242.
My best wishes to you and Tim.
Talk to you soon.
As your shirt says – I'll be multi-tasking on Sat. haha
Jon

To: JonFrankel
Subject: RE: Leaving it.....

Cool! We will definitely be watching. What hotel are you in.. and how long are you staying to recover... er vacation... before you come home?
P.S. I know this sounds goofy... and the last thing you need is 11th hour advice... but my trainer gave me this...When you are tired and you feel like your legs can't take another step... take some deep even breaths and tell yourself you are breathing oxygen into the muscles in your legs... picture it going in. (no I'm not smoking anything) OK stop rolling your eyes.. it works! Just in case though, carry cab fare
Donna

I logged out of my e-mail and into my journal page, grabbing a fistful of tissues from a box on my desk.

Donna's Journal
Home > Health
October 18 , 2002

Hi Folks!

Man... I've got a nasty cold this week. For those of you who tune in... this is not news. Seems to have settled right in my voice. I guess some people might think that's a good thing. :) If you can't get her to stop talking one way... Really though... I feel fine... just a little hoarse. Anyone with a remedy for that... I'd love to hear from you!

If you are counting down with me... and I hope you are... I only have two more chemo treatments! Wow... these are the longest couple of weeks... but with a smile. I've been thinking about all the things I want to do when I'm done.

Since I finish on Halloween I think I should do the shows dressed as a bald woman with no eyelashes... WELL... I should get to choose my Halloween costume shouldn't I?

Once my stomach gets off the drug roller coaster... I'm going to eat everything I want... and a lot of it... and if I get sick... well at least it will be of my own making!

I am going to run until my legs fall off.

I'm going to wrestle my 7-year-old son and WIN.

I'm going to let my daughter teach me all her cool new jump rope moves.

And I am going to stay as far away from needles as humanly possible!

And that's just the first day!!!

Hope I gave you a smile... you give me one every day. As always, have a great week and God bless.

Donna

It was so much easier for me to make jokes than to try to share the dark side with people. I was trying hard not to go there myself. Plus, just writing down all those things I could do when I was finished brightened the gloom. As did the e-mails I received in return.

To: donnahicken@firstcoastnews.com
Subject: 'from Donna's Journal'

Hey Donna,

I love your halloween "no hair" idea. It appeals to my sense of humor. Someone gave me a T-shirt that says "I've used all my sick days so I'm calling in dead." I have it put away with instructions to put it on me when I ever (not for a long long time) die. People will walk by my coffin and say "she hasn't changed a bit. Still going for the laugh."

Anyway, though I have not written before, just want you to know that I have been keeping up with you and praying

and believing that God has good and great things in store for you.
Best wishes, love and prayers,
Shirley Trapp

To: donnahicken@firstcoastnews.com
Subject: 'from Donna's Journal'

Hey, Donna! I just read your Journal entry for this week. And, yes! I am counting down with you!!! I meant to write earlier this week and let you know how much you are in my thoughts. I went through chemo during this time of year, too and the weather this week has brought back those memories and feelings in full force! I also have a nasty cold this week which isn't easy for a Music teacher. :)
As for Halloween costumes... I used the "bald woman" costume and had my husband draw a face on the back of my head so... when I went to the door to open it to the kids, their eyes got really BIG! And then I turned my back on them to get the candy and they saw the face on the back of my head, too! It was a blast!!! Gives new meaning to "eyes in the back of your head." :) It was the one day I could let it all go and not worry about what anyone else might think or feel about my bald and beautiful head!!!
Hang in there!
Rhonda Gauger

To: donnahicken@firstcoastnews.com
Subject: Sore Throat

1. Echinacea tea, does wonders. Both for the throat and for the immune system. It also fights bacterial and viral infections.

2. Vitamin C -has antiviral properties take 5,000 to 20,000 mg a day (not all at once) they have throat drops with vitamin C and Zinc. They are the best. (the zinc tastes like crap though). You can dissolve vitamin C powder in water or juice and sip it to sooth the throat.

3. Garlic (Kyolic) take 2 capsules 3 times a day, for improved immune function

4. Multivitamin and mineral complex, it is important to maintain a balance of all necessary nutrients.

5. Raspberry leaf tea is good for easing the pain of a sore throat as well as fever blisters.

6. Gargle with sea salt solution, 1/2 teaspoon salt in a glass of warm water.

7. Use a mixture of raw honey and lemon juice to coat and soothe the throat.

8. It is usually a good idea to sanitize your toothbrush between brushes when you have a sore throat. You can use hydrogen peroxide, (make sure you rinse well before brushing) or you can use grapefruit seed extract to kill the germs.

Hope you get to feeling better. :o)
Our prayers are with you
Dorinda Kline (Middleburg, FL)

That weekend we tracked Jon on the computer. The weather was stormy just before the race and the waves were churning when the athletes started the swim. My nerves were on edge. I can't imagine what Jon must have been feeling. It was wild to wait for the results, then follow his number as he moved from the swim to the bike. It took forever for the computer to update the final transition. I started to wonder if Jon had quit.

"We should have seen his number by now," I told Tim.

"Sometimes it just takes a while. Be patient. He'll be there."

The computer became the watched pot that never boils. I finally just left it for a while and when I came back there he was.

Number 242 was multi-tasking his way to the finish. He had been dreading the marathon. His knees were killing him. He just wanted to survive it. And he did. Jon didn't set any land speed records, but despite the fact that his knees had other ideas, he finished.

I felt a momentary rush of optimism.

"My knees felt like they were coming off at about mile six," he told me that night on the phone. "I'll never do it again."

"People always say that Jon. Give yourself a few days and I bet you'll feel differently."

"Not a chance," he said. "I'll just come watch you when you do yours."

"I already have done mine," I thought.

Almost anyway.

It's difficult to describe my feelings halfway through that vicious last month of chemo. Literally, because I think I blocked so much of it out. The POW in survival mode. I wanted to be brave. I wanted to be that positive person everyone was talking about. And sometimes I was. The support helped so much. I just couldn't go too deep. My journal entries had become very surface. In one I simply relayed my "Faith" passage word for word. But it wasn't insincere. That's how I was living. On the surface. I couldn't look at myself for more than the couple of minutes it took me to get my make-up on at work. I felt horrible that Tim had to look at me. Although to his credit, he never treated me one ounce different. I had the most difficulty looking at my children. I was convinced some days that I was going to die and that they would be left to deal with it. To live their lives without me. And what would happen to me? I pictured my body. I worried about my soul. I prayed for strength. I prayed for grace. I prayed that God would take my fear away.

"This is all perfectly normal," Edith reminded me almost daily.

But normal was no longer a word I could understand. There was no such thing.

"Just get through this minute Donna," I told myself. "This second."

"Move your right foot in front of your left." But I was sleepwalking.

As with any pressure building just under the surface, eventually it was going to blow.

One night Dan, my former husband, was trying to lighten my mood with a joke about my cancer. Dan is one of the funniest people on the planet and he can always make me laugh. Not this night. I went off on him, sobbing frantically.

"You think I'm going to die don't you," I screamed.

"Donna, come on, I was just kidding, you're going to be fine, come on now."

"I can't do this anymore, Dan. I can't take it."

"Yes, you can. You're just tired. Stop now."

"I need you to believe I'm going to live, Dan," I pleaded. "Maybe more than any other person in the world."

"You're going to live, Donna. Of course you're going to live."

I desperately needed for the father of my children to believe I was going to be there to raise them. As if somehow his thinking it would make it true.

Despite all of the hurt between us, Dan has often been a friend to me. He has a confidence about his words that is contagious. I wanted to be infected with that confidence.

I was hanging on by the tiniest thread, and that thread was unraveling.

To add insult to injury I had received a horribly insensitive e-mail from a woman who was "concerned" that I was letting myself go and asked why I didn't make the effort to wear some make-up and look decent.

"Come on, Donna," she wrote. "I don't think you are even trying."

If that woman could have seen me without the mounds of make-up I applied every day, she would have probably fainted.

"Do you really think I want to look like this?" I wrote back.

When I signed off the air at 11:35 that night I was crashing.

"Are you sure you can drive home?" Tim asked.

It was one of those rare nights when we had to take two cars to work. Tim was planning to follow me home to make sure I stayed awake.

"I'll be OK," I said. "Just honk at me if I fall asleep."

Tim drives like an old man. No, slower. I had lost him in traffic a few miles into the trip.

My eyelids were coming down hard. My head jerked back violently each time they closed.

"Stay awake girl, just a little farther." I told myself. I blasted the air conditioner. I popped in a favorite U-2 CD and cranked it, wailing to heaven along with Bono the lead singer. "isolation, desolation..... let it gooo.... I'm wide awaaaaaaake, I'm wide awaaaaaaaake, I'm wide awaaaaaake, I'm not sleeping." The song is a desperate plea, a release.

As I screamed the words, I started to cry, then shake. The whole world was closing in on me. I was only three blocks from home and I had to pull the car over. I hadn't had a panic attack for years, but this was one for the ages.

"Stop it, Donna! Stop, stop, stop!" I tried to out-scream the terror in my head.

"Dear Jesus, help me," I sobbed. "I've lost the handle Lord. Do you hear me? I can't hold on. You've got to catch me. I'm falling. Please Jesus, please."

I don't know how long I sat there racked with tears begging for help. Probably no more than five minutes, but it took every bit of strength I had left to crank the ignition and turn the steering wheel for home.

As it turns out Jesus was listening. So was His Mother. And fortunately for me, so was a very devout man named Jeff.

I arrived at work the next day to find a miracle, disguised as the

151

torn corner of a piece of notebook paper, on my desk. On it, was scribbled these words.

"Donna –
Jeff called at 4:37 this morning. Says he needs to talk with you as soon as possible."

Jeff's phone number was at the bottom.

"4:37," I said. "That's weird."

I tracked down the person who left the note, and sure enough, the time was right.

I sat down at my desk and dialed the number. Jeff answered.

"Donna, first of all I want you to know I am not crazy," he said.

"Well, that makes one of us," I replied.

"My name is Jeff McCrory. We've never met. I created the shrine to The Virgin Mary at St. Paul's and I'm working to complete the one over at the Catholic radio station."

"I've seen both, they're beautiful," I said. But my mind was starting to race.

"Something has happened and I want to share it with you."

I could feel my heart pounding in my chest.

"Is this something good, or something bad?" I asked, my voice cracking.

"Something very good," he said. Jeff's voice was shaking too. We were both on the verge of tears.

"You called just after 4:30 this morning," I said. "What is it, what's happened?"

"I need to see you in person. Can we meet at the shrine in front of the radio station?"

The request took me by surprise. It's something I would normally never do. There are many beautiful people out there with great intentions.

I learned quickly in this business, there are also a handful who

152

could do me harm.

"OK," I said. "How about tomorrow morning?"

"See you then."

Tim went with me.

When we got to the radio station, Jeff met us outside. We introduced ourselves and then Jeff and I walked over by the shrine.

As Catholics we hold the Mother of Christ in high regard. In the gospel of John chapter 19 Jesus is dying on the cross. He sees His Mother and the apostle John and says to Mary, "Woman, behold thy son" and to John "behold thy mother." Catholics believe that as followers of Jesus, Mary became the mother of the church and of us all. We do not in any way put her on par with Jesus, or suggest that we need to take our prayers to another. We turn to her in prayer much the same way many of us turn to loved ones who are in heaven for strength and intercession.

"My whole life I've been praying to Mary," Jeff said. "I ask that if there is anyone I can help, anyone I can comfort, please let me know. I've prayed this for years and I have never received a specific direction. That changed yesterday morning."

Tears started to well in my eyes.

"Just after 4 a.m., I woke up to see The Virgin Mary standing at the foot of my bed. You were standing next to her."

Jeff paused for a moment.

"I'm telling you Donna, I'm as sane as they get, and I know the difference between a dream and reality and this was no dream. It happened. I wasn't thinking about you or praying for you or anything. And there you were with Mary."

"What did she say?"

"She didn't speak. I just had the immediate sense that I was supposed to call you right then and there and let you know that everything is going to be all right. So if there is anything that has been troubling you, or if you have been praying for anything in particular, it's going to be OK. And I wanted to give you this."

Jeff reached into his pocket and handed me a scapular. It had a necklace-like chain and a piece of felt at either end with images of

153

The Virgin Mary. Much like a rosary, it is simply a tool to help us focus in on our prayer life.

Jeff and I both cried and hugged.

"I can't tell you what a gift this is Jeff."

"For me too," he said. "If I never talk to you again after today, I've done what I was supposed to do."

I knew what he meant. I never told Jeff about my panic attack or my plea to God. I didn't have to.

I ran to the car and poured the story out to Tim. We cried all the way back home.

I was anxious to tell my mom. Before the chemo, I often prayed the rosary while I was running, but my mother says it in her sleep.

Her response wasn't exactly what I expected, but in hindsight it makes sense.

"Why wouldn't The Virgin Mary just come directly to you, Donna? Why would she go to someone else?"

For all of her faith in God, my mother is the first to tell you she has a fatal flaw. She loves God, no doubt. But it's that 'love thy neighbor' thing she has a tough time with.

"It's the one thing that's going to keep me out of heaven," she laments.

"God is great, but I can't stand his people."

"We are supposed to be here to minister to each other Mom," I said.

"We're the body of Christ, together. Don't you see? It's beautiful. We both received a gift."

It was like that with my e-mails too. Each e-mail was that communion between people. People gave me courage and hope, and somehow I returned it to them.

TEN

Trick or Treat?

I wanted to share my miracle with the journal readers, but I hesitated. It was one thing to talk about God and prayer on a company website, but telling people I'd received this incredible gift from the Mother of Christ was quite another. I didn't doubt its authenticity, I simply didn't want to overstep my bounds. More though, I didn't want to offend those of other beliefs. My faith is my own. I've given it tremendous thought and test, and care. It's not possible for anyone else to share the exact same faith. Faith, or lack of it for that matter, is intensely personal.

And there was something else. The message was that "everything would be all right." What that meant exactly, I didn't know.

"It may have absolutely nothing to do with the cancer," I told Tim, as we went over the conversation for the hundredth time. "We could be talking about a much bigger picture."

On the small screen of my daily life, there were still many other things to share. I kept my miracle to myself.

Donna's Journal
Home > Health
October 28, 2002

Hi Folks!
So many nice notes from you about my countdown. Thank you so very much for the continued love, support

155

and encouragement. I will never be able to convey to you adequately how much you have and do lift me.

Can you believe it's been six months since I shared my re-diagnosis with you? Along the way I have made so many new friends.... felt so many prayers. You've put up with me while I've tried to laugh and occasionally cried.... and you've done those things with me.

I have so many mixed emotions about my last treatment this week. On the one hand... I'm thrilled beyond words to be finishing chemo. It's been such a long haul physically and emotionally. I'm ready to look like myself again... pixie head and all! I'm ready to feel like I'm 41 instead of 141!

But I'm also scared to pieces. For those of you who have been here ... you will understand. The thought of not actively doing something to "fight back" is frightening. I went for my blood work last week...and one of the nurses congratulated me. Purely out of her excitement she said... "before you know it... you'll be back for your follow up tests and that'll be that." It was all I could do to make it to the car before I just lost it. The thought of those tests is so unnerving.

Anyhow... those are passing worries...that must do just that... pass. It's useless to obsess about such things... yet from time to time... it's just what we do.

I told you at the beginning of this journey that God has a plan for me. I am not in control of that plan. I just try to follow.... without tripping myself up any more than I am bound to do!

I'll give you the big thumbs up when I get through this week... and after that I will keep you updated on some plans that I hope will make a difference in this fight for others.

God bless all of you... and have a great week!!!
Donna

To: donnahicken@firstcoastnews.com
Subject: Thanks

Donna...
Thank you for answering my e-mail... kinda surprised me... but a nice surprise... knowing how busy you are... well... you're a MOM... that should say it all... LOL
I think the thing that scares me... are the little things that I think don't bother me... but truly do... like today, being my 15 yr old's birthday... I want to see more of them... and her graduation... college... marriage... and of course, her kids... I want to see it ALL.... (how selfish... huh??)
I know God has a plan for all of this... and He will get the glory out of all of this... but I keep sticking my chin out and saying... "OK, God... now what??"
I keep praying that you will never have to deal with this demon (cancer) again... cause that's what it is... it steals the life right out of you... sometimes... in such a short time...
Forgive me for asking... but I have already decided... I don't want a lumpectomy... I want a mastectomy... 'cause it's in my lymphnodes also... here's the question... did they do a lumpectomy on you... or a mastectomy... forgive me for being too honest... but I have been doing my homework and looking up anything I can find on breast

157

cancer and I know from reading article after article... that having a lumpectomy only... means a greater chance of it coming back... I know a mastectomy doesn't mean total protection... but I need to be around for my 6-month-old's fifth birthday... I am determined to have as much control over my "disease" as I possibly can...

Thank you again... and many blessing's on your last treatment on Thursday...YEAH!!!!!!

Be blessed...

Andee Ryan

To: AndeeRyan
Subject: RE: Thanks

Hi Andee,

I understand how you feel about the mastectomy. Although much of the recent research shows virtually no difference in the two... if I had it to do all over again... that's exactly what I would have done. I had a lumpectomy. I think you should follow your gut.

It will likely give you more peace of mind. Besides they can make you a new one that you may even like better!! I pray that you will be there for many many more birthdays... weddings... grandchildren etc... Just take the days one at a time. You'll get through it. I'm scared too... but you can't let the fear rule you or you won't enjoy those good times with your kids. I'm not sure anyone who has had cancer ever quite looks at life the same again... but maybe we have a greater appreciation. Hang in there girl and take care.

Donna

To: donnahicken@firstcoastnews.com
Subject: 'from Donna's Journal'

I work at the Duval County Courthouse, and over the years, I've been drawn to watching you, keeping up with your life, etc. I was so especially surprised to discover your journal today. During lunch, there are such few places to go that are in the vicinity of the Courthouse, I find myself eating yogurt, and surfing the web, or reading. I found a cancer support group on the internet, which I've enjoyed participating in, when I have the opportunity. I do not have cancer, but I was a care giver of my Mom and Grandfather at the same time. My Mom died last year of lymphoma non-Hodgkins, and my Grandfather died 6 weeks later of colon/prostate cancer. My best friend was diagnosed with breast cancer right after that, and is currently undergoing basically the same things you are right now.

I found myself having nightmares about cancer. Paranoid and petrified that I would too, someday contract this horrible disease. Little by little, I have been able to overcome this fear. I'm a Judicial Assistant for one of the Circuit Judges, and we are currently on the Family Law bench, and have been for over three years. We see horrible cases each and every day, people fighting over the most petty of issues, i.e., who gets the broken VCR, who gets who's retirement accounts, etc.

Once I experienced death from a personal view, it has seemed to put the rest of life into perspective. I am a 42 year old woman, who now, goes home and kisses and hugs my daughters (I have four, ages 22 to 11), hugs and kisses my Husband (all of a sudden his dirty laundry in the floor seems to not matter anymore), and I come into work with a love for and zest for life. One that I don't believe I ever had before. I know how difficult it is to share personal feelings about something like this, and I just am thankful to have the opportunity to tell you how much I admire you, your courage and strength throughout this entire ordeal. What a ministry of helping others through your experience. For the first time, I can now view what I've been through personally in my life as a blessing. The Lord has taught me many lessons throughout this experience - not to take life for granted, the little things really don't matter all that much, and tell people how you feel about them NOW, while you have the opportunity, and last but not least, my messy house can WAIT! Thank you Donna, for allowing your life to be so visible to others. Thank you for sharing your marriage, divorce, childbirths, illnesses, and all other aspects of your life with a public audience whom you don't know. You have touched my life, inspired me to be a stronger woman, and to rally around those that need me.

God Bless you always -
Love Lisa Chacon

To: LisaChacon
Subject: RE: 'from Donna's Journal'

Hi Lisa,
What a beautiful letter. Thank you so much for your kind words and for sharing that with me. It means more than I can tell you. As a girl raised in Catholic school... I am well acquainted with guilt and worry! But you're right, there is something about facing something that could potentially take your life... or the lives of those you love, that changes your perspective. It's really too bad everyone can't get the appreciation without necessarily going through the fear. Sounds like family law has a good person on its side. I know those folks need you! God bless you

and thanks again for taking the time to share your thoughts with me. It's people like you who really lift me on days when I'm feeling puny. Take care.
Donna

"Who needs Halloween candy," I thought. The words were sweeter and more satisfying than any candy could ever be.

The day before my final treatment, I sat at the dining room table and contemplated the deep subject of Halloween candy. Being the chocoholic I am, I usually raid the kids' candy bags the moment they come home from trick or treat.

"Maybe Baby Ruth," I thought. "Snickers?" I was calculating the odds. Which of these was less likely to make me puke.

"Beware the Ninja," Drew shrieked, jumping out from behind the counter, his sword drawn.

"Drew-dog you scared me to death," I said. "Don't you want to save your costume for tomorrow night?"

"Just trying it on Mom. Do I look mean?"

Drew's doe-like brown eyes and mile-long eyelashes flashed from behind his glasses.

"The meanest," I said, wanting to eat him up with a spoon. "Try not to poke someone's eye out with that sword."

"Mom, it's plastic."

"Really, and I thought it was solid steel."

"That's called sarcasm right?" Drew cocked his head and cut me a sideways look.

"Very good my love, learn from the master."

"Are you really going to go on the air bald for Halloween?"

"Do you think I should?"

"You might be scarier than me."

"Yes, I might," I laughed. "Would it bother you if I did it?"

"Gosh no, Mom. I can't wait for all my friends to see my mother's shiny head on the news."

I narrowed my gaze on the Ninja before me. "That's sarcasm

161

right?"

Drew threw me an exaggerated grin.

I knew I'd never do it. Even though a lot of viewers were egging me on. The station management had twisted and turned with me through every crazy gyration. I wasn't about to push things any further. But I was tempted.

Halloween was never one of my favorite holidays. It's too dark for me. This year it was Independence Day. Of course independence comes with its own challenges. Still, I couldn't wait to rip off that wig. Realistically I knew it would be months before my own hair was long enough to wear on the air. I was just aching to be myself. Whoever "myself" was after all of this.

The phone rang.

"Hey there, it's me." My standard salutation from Julie.

"Hi Jules, what's up?"

"Are you getting excited about the grand finale?"

"The chemo?"

"No, the office Halloween party. Of course the chemo."

"I can't wait to be done. But it's sort of like that day in 8th grade with Sister Patrick."

"What?"

Sister Patrick was a nun's nun. Small and compact, she walked like a soldier in the military, her habit flying like a flag from her head. She had a sense of humor to match.

"Remember, we were reading that book, "All's Quiet on the Western Front?"

Sister Patrick chose me to read aloud to the class. As I was going along, I came across the word "helluva".... Something like, "that was a helluva thing to do."

Julie started laughing. It was a classic moment in Catholic education.

"What in the world does this have to do with your final chemo treatment?"

"Remember what she said? She slapped her ruler down on the desk, trained her Irish eyes on me and said 'MISS Hazouri, that word is Hahl-YOU-vah. Say it please.'

"That was a Hahl-YOU-vah thing to do?" I repeated the words trying with every fiber of my being not to laugh. The class erupted, and that was it. I was gone. Detention."

Julie and I were howling at the memory.

"I still don't see what…."

"No win situation," I said. "I insist on pronouncing the word correctly, I'm disrespectful. I pronounce it wrong, and laugh, I'm disrespectful. Detention either way."

The end of chemo was much like that. I was so happy to say goodbye to this vile intrusion, but at least while the drugs were inside my veins they were standing guard. After tomorrow I was on my own. Physical prison, or mental, either prospect was frightening.

Sleep was rarely a problem during chemo. I would collapse in an exhausted heap at the end of the day, and wake in practically the same exact spot. The night before my final treatment I lay blinking in the dark. Every sound was magnified. The steady rumble of the ocean, the clock on the wall, Tim's breathing. The sounds of my world. I wanted so much to take them for granted again.

"Look who's up." Tim smiled over his morning coffee as I walked into the living room.

"Guess I'm a little jazzed. I didn't sleep much."

Tim motioned to the calendar. It was filled with lines. For as long as I can remember, he has made a line through the date at the end of each day. The word "drips" appeared on the only unmarked date left, October 31st.

Drips was our word for chemo.

"I don't want to see THAT word on my calendar every week," I told him at the beginning.

Drips seemed less intimidating.

Underneath the date, the word FINAL jumped from the page.

"Whaddaya say we find something less exciting to do next week," I said.

"Nice and boring," Tim said. "I promise."

Stepping onto the eighth floor of the Mayo Clinic I looked at the familiar faces around me.

"Last one, right?" The woman behind the check-in desk was beaming.

"Last one," I repeated.

"Well, we're gonna miss you around here."

I smiled. That one I couldn't repeat.

"I thought maybe you guys would dress up for me," I said. "It IS Halloween."

"Guess you got the trick instead of the treat today, huh?"

"Both I suppose."

"Well, they're ready for you. Val's waiting to take you back."

I barely turned and Valerie, a tall, beautiful African American nurse had me swept up in a big bear hug.

"You look so good," she gushed. "I'm so happy for you."

I did not look good. In fact I looked decidedly bad, but I appreciated the sentiment.

Feeling the cool liquids drip into my body that last day, I couldn't help but think back to my first diagnosis.

The final treatment was on my 39th birthday. February 28th, 2000. I was surrounded by my dearest friends. There were balloons and presents from the nurses. Edith was there smiling from ear to ear. Aurora was dancing the Macarena and whirling around the room. My friend, and at that time, colleague, Kim Sadler taped the whole thing for the station. It was a party. A cake proclaimed "NO MO CHEMO." I felt giddy and confident, and thankful. Most of all I felt done.

"Where are you?" Tim's question brought me back to the present.

"Exactly where I was two and a half years ago," I said.

But it was in location only. I didn't feel any of those strong emotions now. I was thankful to be alive. Relieved to be stepping across the finish line. Comforted by a new vision that on some level things would all work out as they should. Beyond that I hadn't a clue in the world.

"You'll get your confidence back, Donna," a nurse named Vicki had told me. "You get a few good tests behind you, and you'll see things turn around."

"Spoken with the conviction of someone who has never had the anguish of post-chemo blood work," I thought.

A loud beep signaled the medicine had dripped it's last drop. The end of the race. My legs could rest. At least for now.

"One, two, three and we're out," the nurse said as she removed the needle from my chest for the final time.

I took a deep breath and a smile spread across my face.

"You made it," Tim said pulling me into an embrace.

"We made it," I corrected him.

Tim had gone with me to every treatment. He had watched me giggle with my Benadryl, gasp for air during my allergic reaction, cry out of sheer nervous energy. He had fetched blankets when I was cold and cold cloths when I was hot. He listened to every insane thought in my bald head and treated me like the most beautiful woman in the world.

"My work here is done," I said, mockingly waving a dismissive hand to the nursing station. "Find someone else to torture."

Hugs descended on me from around the room.

You will never convince me that chemo nurses aren't truly angels in disguise. The pain they see and so often the slow march to death is daily fare. Even patients who survive, undergo the inevitable transformation before their eyes. Someone enters their realm full of color and energy and life. They watch it all slowly ebb away to the shell. Some grotesque horror movie where humans become zombies. Yet, if there is one word to describe every chemo nurse I have ever met, it is "optimistic." Genuinely optimistic. Yes, they are compassionate, caring, nurturing, all the things you would expect from professional caregivers. But what cancer patients need more than all of that is for someone to believe they can make it.

A lot of people give lip service to that belief. But the vacant

165

look always gives them away. That, "Oh thank God it's not me" look. The very people who have every reason to hang the vacancy sign never give in to that.

They believe.

My angels on the eighth floor always came through.

*　　*　　*

"Coming through." First Coast News photographer Jim McIntyre announced his presence, as he lugged his camera equipment past me and into the photog lounge.

The spot where the anchors have to stand to tease the next newscast almost blocks the way to their door. So the photographers have to wait for the right time, then dash across when the "on air" light goes off.

As Jim passed, he squeezed my arm. Everyone knew this was a big day for me. Jim flashed a grin. He and I had been forced to bond.

During the 2000 presidential election we thought we were being sent to Tallahassee for the dramatic "end" to a very tight race between George W. Bush and Al Gore. Jim, our satellite truck operator Eric Decker, and another photographer Mark Vandiver, worked around the clock. We were in a tiny truck. We ate very bad food. We made impossible deadlines. It was great! Every adrenaline junkie's dream.

I was in my element.

If I have a strength as a reporter, it is this. I don't need time to memorize lines. I don't even want to, it just messes me up. Just give me the information. Let me process it in my brain, and I will simply talk to the viewers about what I know.

I think I have the ability to take a lot of clutter, boil it down to its essence and give it back.

This doesn't always sit well with the producers back at the station.

"I need a roll cue for your bite, Donna."

A bite is just news lingo for sound. A ten second piece of an interview is a bite.

Producers and directors like to have a roll cue, your last words before the interview. If they know what you are going to say, they know when to roll the bite.

"I don't know what I'm going to say, I'll just make it obvious."

Silence.

"OK."

It may sound lazy, but it really isn't. If I try to memorize something and forget my exact words, I get that deer in the headlights look that you have no doubt seen on reporter's faces when they lose their train of thought.

Besides, I think if people have a comfort level with me, it is because I just talk to them. Not at them. I don't rehearse a speech I just have a conversation.

It was a mad dash to the finish for every live report.

The principals in my stories were like characters in a play.

James Baker, the former Secretary of State under Ronald Reagan would deliver the daily spin from the Republican side. He had the appearance of a proud eagle perched at the lectern, quiet and poised. For the Democrats it was Warren Christopher. Christopher was Jimmy Carter's Deputy Secretary of State, known for his role in negotiating an end to the Iran hostage crisis. He was later Secretary of State under Bill Clinton.

We called him "the human coat hanger."

I have never seen anyone so thin in my entire life. When he turned sideways he would practically disappear. And he wore a sour expression on his face, as if he were perpetually smelling something rotten. Perhaps he already knew something about how things would turn out for his Party's candidate.

Thirty-seven days, hundreds of stories and live reports, and thousands of hanging chads later, it was finally over. After weeks of lower court decisions, and threats from the Florida Legislature, the election was decided by the U.S. Supreme Court. George W. Bush was the nations 43rd president.

It was the most work and the most fun I have ever had as a journalist.

We had arrived weeks before Thanksgiving, along with throngs of national and international press. We left amidst the twinkle of Christmas lights strung across the scores of satellite trucks that made the journey. We witnessed history together. We were part of history. The moment was even more profound for me. I was alive to see it, having just come back to life from my first introduction to chemotherapy.

"First Coast News Anchor Donna Hicken joins us now, with more on what we can expect tonight at 11, Donna." Alan tossed it to me from the set.

I read my tease, but as I was talking, I began to feel an uneasy churning in my stomach. Too early for the chemo to be rearing it's ugly head. It was nerves. I knew that night I would tell people that my chemo was over. Tell them, not in the journal, but on the air. I felt a sudden pang of insecurity. The journal had become my only comfort zone in sharing my disease.

Later, when I logged on to my e-mail, I was reminded of why it was so.

To: donnahicken@firstcoastnews.com
Subject: 'from Donna's Journal'

Hi Donna,

I have been reading your journal entries, but have hesitated to 'write'. There is so much that I have wanted to say to you, but I worried that I might say the wrong thing. So please know that I send these words to you out of a sense of love and encouragement.

First of all, let me say how proud of you I am. Having experienced cancer through family members and close friends, I do have some idea of what you have been going through.

I lost my Mom to breast cancer when I was 14 years old, after she had valiantly fought a 10-year fight. I dare say that if she were diagnosed today, I'd still have my Mom around. I know that sometimes it must be hard for you to count blessings, but please do know that you have so much more available to you now than my Mom did.

My niece from Key West was diagnosed with lymphoma just over five years ago. I was fortunate enough to be able to quickly get her into Mayo for treatment. They told her that they had never seen a mass as large as hers. She basically lived with me on-and-off while she was having chemo. When she was first diagnosed, she had 3 kids under age 4, and during her ordeal, she and her husband divorced. What a shame he was not man enough to be there for her when she really needed the support of family. But - she is truly a success story. When she returns in February for her follow-up visit, she will have been in successful remission for over 5 years! I am so grateful for her caregivers at Mayo!

What have I learned from these two very strong and courageous women?... to fight like hell. I know that you know it's a battle - it's a battle that must be ferociously fought. I also know that you must allow your body and your soul some leeway for the battle that you have been and are still going through.

As I reread what I've written you, I realize that what I've said is most assuredly nothing that you do not already know. Except, perhaps, that there is one more person 'out here' that's in your corner, celebrating with and for you every victory, no matter how small or large, and sending you lots of love and encouragement. I further hope and pray that you realize how much love and encouragement others in your circumstances are receiving by your sharing of your experiences. Maybe on one of those days when you're too exhausted to lift a single finger, or you're just hurting inside and out, and you're wondering why - maybe you'll know that even through this whole experience God was able to use it for good - through the love and encouragement others have received through you.

God bless you Donna!

Sincerely,

Sandy Bernreuter

"How do you want to do this?" Alan asked as we planned the newscast.

"Let's do it on the toss to weather," I said. "That way, we can make quick mention of it, and be done."

I knew once again, my preferred method of communication on the issue wouldn't be my news director's choice, but to his credit, he always left that call up to me.

"We need to congratulate Donna on a big day," Alan told the viewers at 11.

"Yes, I've finished my last day of chemo, hopefully, the last time we'll be talking about me and chemo in the same sentence."

"Definitely the last time," Tim added.

"Thank all of you so much for your prayers and support," I said, turning to the camera. "Now, let's talk about the weather."

And that was that.

I will confess to you in all humility that I am usually completely comfortable on the air. I can imagine I'm in a room with friends, talking. Being on the anchor desk is the least stressful part of what

I do. That night, I felt like a cub reporter, sweating her first live interview.

On the drive home, I was ready for sleep. The last ghosts and goblins darted across the road as we pulled into the neighborhood.

"It's good to be home," Tim said, turning the key in the lock.

I kicked off my shoes, walked to the sliding glass door and pulled it open.

"The ocean's still there," I called back to Tim as I took a deep cleansing breath of salt air.

"Want to do the honors?" he asked, pointing to the calendar.

"No please, go right ahead."

Tim drew a line through October 31st.

"Thank you Lord," he said.

"Amen."

The hallelujah chorus from Donna's Journal began immediately.

To: donnahicken@firstcoastnews.com
Subject: 'from Donna's Journal'

Hi Donna — I'm Donna too! :-)
I've been reading your journal and, of course, watching you on TV.....
I don't know if I can quite put into words how I'm feeling..... I don't have cancer and I won't pretend to understand everything you've been through...... I have my own mess of issues to deal with and oh how I envy your courage!!
I know you've been afraid. Who wouldn't be? But I've watched you go through this valley with your head up & and your hands stretched out to God. I know you've cried. Who wouldn't? But yet I watch your beautiful smile and listen for the humor in your journal.
The beauty inside you shines through.
Thank you for being open and sharing your illness with

us. I've prayed for you so many times and I'm trusting that God will lead you all the way out of the valley.

I also want to thank you for the passage you shared from the book you've been reading, "Living Faith." I've read and reread it. What a blessing!! I'd like to know who wrote the book because I'd like to get one. I tried to find it online but there are so many with the same title that I thought I'd better ask you. If you want to post it on the website that would be great.

Today is the last day of chemo and the first day of the rest of your life. Go get 'em Donna!!

God bless you

Donna Grover

To: donnahicken@firstcoastnews.com
Subject: 'from Donna's Journal'

Hi Donna

Just want to say CONGRAT'S, CONGRATS, CONGRATS.

I sound like Gomer Pyle, well anyway this is a day early because I knew tomorrow your e-mail would be full. I'm so proud of you I think you are one brave person.

I would like to wish you all the luck in the world, although I don't think you are going to need it as I just know this monster is gone for good!

I am reading a very good book you might be interested in, called "The Magic of Believing" by Claude M. Bristol, It really gets you thinking.

Well Happy Halloween I know it will be one you will always remember. Hopefully we can meet one day!

Until then remember there are only Tomorrow's and no yesterday's.

Sincerely

Janice Schiebler

ELEVEN

Brain Freeze

Donna's Journal
Home > Health
November 4 , 2002

Hi Folks!

As I write this I am still feeling that lovely hangover that only chemotherapy can provide... but that's OK. I can look at it now and say in a few days... I'll feel better... and then in a few more days...better still. No bags of "goodies" waiting for me next week. WWAAAAAHOOOOO!

I mentioned my final treatment on the air last Friday...and it made me realize how much more comfortable I have become writing in this journal. It's just so hard for me to talk about this stuff on the air. It seems inappropriate somehow... I don't know... I just know it's tough for me to do. Many of you have asked if I could continue the journal... and I will on some level. More to come on that when I get it all figured out.

I have often told you how much your prayers and support have and do mean to me. I haven't however talked much about the folks here... and I want to share with you how important they have been in making it possible for me to keep working through all this craziness.

My bosses let me come in late... rest between shows... basically whatever I needed to be able to hold my head up and talk to you in the evenings. My co-anchors have picked up the slack for me when I was too sick to come in...and my producers have put up with my chemo-brain! Six months is a long time. Anyhow I just wanted you to know that I work with some pretty incredible folks... who have been awfully good to me.

I have often alluded to helping others who are dealing with this disease. Toward that end... I am (with enormous help) organizing a foundation to help women who have difficulty affording treatment. No one should have a better prognosis than anyone else because of money. I had hoped to have everything up and running by now... but the truth is I was just too pooped to put in the necessary time. The framework is in place... now I just need to get moving. I will... of course keep you updated on that.

As far as my health is concerned... I sure hope and pray that my role in this disease is now limited to helping others. No matter what the future holds... I know fighting this disease will always be a part of my life. For those of you who are battling or have family battling cancer... please know that I am here to listen or to help in any way I can.

I hope I will continue to hear from you. As far as I'm concerned we're family.

Have a great week and God bless! As always, your biggest fan.

Donna

As I typed the last words of that November 4th journal entry, I felt a wave of sadness. I was ready to move on. Ready to put cancer behind me. Ready to have my life back. But what was my life? Certainly not what it was before. I was in a new family now. I knew it when I was first diagnosed, but the journal really brought it home. Fighting cancer is as much a part of me as anchoring the news.

I had this disease for a reason.

When I was initially diagnosed in 1999 the cancer actually saved my life. I mentioned my week-long stay in the hospital, when my blood counts dropped and the doctors couldn't control my fever. During that week, I began having intense headaches. I was sure it was from all the different antibiotics they were giving me. Edith wanted confirmation.

"I've ordered an MRI of your brain, Donna, just to rule out anything else."

Anything else.

I didn't mention the 'anything else' and neither did she. We both knew what we weren't saying.

I was exhausted from fighting the infection. Just realizing I could see again as the fog of fever and pain dissolved. Maybe I wasn't yet coherent enough to be freaked out. Maybe I was still in that "slam dunk" mentality that told me I would get through this hell and life would be what it was. But aside from my fear of tight spaces, the thought of the test didn't really scare me. I just wanted it over.

"This will only take a few minutes," Edith offered.

I was slipped into a narrow tube that made me feel horribly claustrophobic.

The nurse put a towel over my eyes and that seemed to help. For the next several minutes loud banging and knocking sounds filled the chamber. They would stop for a moment or two, and then start again. Stop then start.

"They must be getting close," I thought. More time ticked by. More banging and knocking.

175

For what seemed like an eternity there was nothing, no sound at all.

Finally, the nurse's voice broke the silence.

"We are going to need a few more pictures Donna, are you OK in there?"

"I want to talk to Edith," I said, "Pull me out of this thing."

This was taking way too long. A few minutes had become the better part of an hour. I had entered this little experiment fully expecting to find nothing wrong. Medicine always gave me headaches. I was starting to doubt my confidence.

The tube gave a slight jolt and began to move. I took the towel from my eyes and squinted, adjusting to the light of the room. Edith was waiting on the outside.

"I'm sorry, you must be worried," she said. " We haven't found anything... horrible."

Edith's pause said more than her words.

"What does THAT mean?" I asked, feeling annoyed that someone didn't just cut to the chase.

"Well, Donna, it seems you have a rather large aneurysm."

An aneurysm, I was told, is a weak spot in a blood vessel. It creates a pocket of blood that, should it burst, would likely be fatal.

I needed brain surgery.

"Brain surgery! Please tell me this is a bad joke."

My life seemed to be one bad joke after another at the moment, and I was not amused.

The aneurysm was nearly nine millimeters in diameter, a dangerous size. It was nestled behind my right eye. The doctors said it was likely it had been there "forever."

I was to talk with Mayo's neurosurgeons about the prospect of cutting through my skull and repairing the blood vessel.

Doctor Ron Reimer was my first consultation. Dr. Reimer has dark wavy hair and a mustache, and a speaking tone that doesn't change whether he's talking about his beautiful children or a patient with a brain tumor. His tone masks his true nature. He is very kind

176

and surprisingly sensitive.

"You definitely need the surgery, Donna. I'm not sure I would wait until after the chemo, but there are other things to consider as well."

There was the possibility that because of the location of the aneurysm, and where the doctors would have to cut, my face could droop on one side after the surgery.

"There goes my career," I thought.

But there was another option: a procedure that would be less invasive and produce the same result, without the worry of disfiguring my face. A brilliant neuroradiologist named David Miller was one of the only doctors in the country who could do it. My first consultation with Dr. Miller was over the phone.

"We'll need to do an angiogram to see exactly what we're dealing with," he said.

Dr. Miller would put a catheter into my femoral artery at the top of my right thigh, shoot dye into my brain to illuminate it, and take a look around.

"Sounds like fun," I said.

"Oh it is."

David Miller and I had an instant rapport. From the moment I first heard his voice, he was someone I knew. I felt totally at ease with him, and completely safe.

"I can trust a man who's as sarcastic as I am," I said.

"Good. I'll see you at the hospital. And don't worry, the shaking stops entirely when I operate."

When I arrived at St. Luke's, they put me in one of those lovely gowns that ties in the back and stuck me in a room where I swear it was so cold I could see my breath.

"Where do they hang the meat in here?" I asked the nurse.

"It has to be cold for all the equipment," she said.

The same is true at the television station. I dress for January in June to keep from suffering hypothermia.

The nurse went to grab some blankets and I looked around the room. White and gray.

"Good morning!" Dr. Miller walked in like he was on a mission.

His appearance was striking. Blue eyes beamed from above his surgical mask. They were offset by his brown hair and smooth almost olive looking skin.

"You need some color in this room. This is not a fun room," I said.

"Don't hurt my feelings," he said. "This is going to be a great time."

"Let me see your hands," I demanded.

Miller stuck out his hand. Steady as a statue.

"Problem is, I operate with this one." His right hand was wobbling over the table.

"I know, it stops when you operate."

He went on to explain again what we were about to do.

"You'll be awake, but try not to move."

"What happens if I move? Never mind. I won't."

I was more worried about the angiogram than the impending surgery. The only other time I had ever had one was when I was preparing to give my father the kidney. I was 18 and never had so much as a toothache before. Doctors shot dye into my back to highlight the area around my kidneys. The pain was incredible, like someone pouring battery acid on my back. I wasn't looking forward to that sensation in my head.

"Take a breath and hold," Dr. Miller instructed.

When I did, the warm dye shot into my brain. I braced, but after only a slight burning sensation, it was gone. This was repeated about a dozen times until Dr. Miller had all the information he needed.

"It looks good, Donna. The opening to the aneurysm is a little wide. It's not perfect, but it will work."

The surgery would require the same basic drill with a seemingly impossible twist. He would once again, go in through my femoral artery. A small tool would snake it's way all the way up to my brain and the aneurysm. Dr. Miller would essentially stuff tiny platinum coils into the aneurysm, rendering it harmless.

178

"Sounds like science fiction," I thought.

"Considering how much you run, and the fact that you've given birth to two children, you are very fortunate this hasn't ruptured," Miller explained.

"Oh yes, very fortunate," I said. "I'm 39, going through chemotherapy for breast cancer, and now I have a brain aneurysm. Who could be luckier than that?"

But in truth I was lucky. The tests showed my aneurysm had never bled. I was right. The headaches I suffered were from the antibiotics. But they prompted Edith to order the MRI of my brain.

"If there are no real symptoms until it ruptures, how do most people find out they have an aneurysm?" I asked.

"Autopsy reports are very useful," came the answer.

The decision on timing was made for me. The operation would have to wait until my strength and my blood counts improved. Months after the chemo.

Of course when the chemo was done, I was raring to get back in my running shoes. In fact my triumphant return from cancer was going to be the New York Marathon. So many people want to run New York, organizers have to hold a lottery. I was chosen.

"A sure sign I'll be able to run," I thought.

Doctor Miller and I had already sparred over this issue.

"I want my life back, David," I snapped during one visit to his office.

"And I want you to have it back, but insisting on running a marathon right after brain surgery is a little over the top, don't you think?"

"Juvenile" was the word Edith used.

Edith is a huge proponent of my running. Studies show exercise helps decrease your cancer chances.

Long distance runners tend to deplete the estrogen in their bodies as well, and estrogen is breast cancer's best friend.

"The more you exercise, the better," she says.

But this time she too thought I was pushing the envelope.

Much to Dr. Miller's dismay I ran six miles on the beach the morning of my brain surgery, arriving at the hospital horribly dehydrated.

"I forgot I wasn't allowed to drink any water after midnight," I confessed sheepishly.

Several bags of IV fluid later David Miller worked his science fiction on my brain to perfection. The surgery was long, almost seven hours. I woke up feeling like I'd been hit by a bus. But my head was working, at least as much as it ever does. The aneurysm was no longer a ticking time bomb.

Dr. Miller won the war over my marathon. My need to prove I was "back" was outweighed by my desire not to be "juvenile."

I would live to run another day.

Like I said, I had cancer for a reason.

But what I learned the second time around, what people taught me through the journal, was that the reason was bigger than me in a way I'd failed to fully grasp the first time.

I sat staring at the smiling image of me wearing my wig at the top of "Donna's Journal".

That small voice in my head was getting louder.

You are here to serve others.

I recalled one of my first conversations with Edith.

"I don't want to be the poster child for this disease," I said, feeling irritated that this cancer thing was getting in the way of my well planned route through life.

"Because of who you are, you are the poster child either way," she replied.

"You can choose to embrace it and be at peace with it, or fight it and be miserable, but either way, you are the news anchor with breast cancer."

I had long since resolved to take up the banner, but the journal showed me how. People needed my help. Not just my words, but my actions.

I had put the wheels in motion for a foundation to help women fighting breast cancer who couldn't make ends meet. Now it was time to hit the accelerator. I knew just where to find the fuel.

"I've got to contact Cynthia Montello," I thought.

Cynthia is a cancer survivor too. She owns an ad agency. We had never met, but from the moment I first hinted at starting a foundation for women with breast cancer she began e-mailing me about the prospect. It was uncanny. As the months passed, if the Foundation even crossed my mind, I would log on to my computer, and there it was. Another e-mail from Cynthia.

To: donnahicken@firstcoastnews.com
Subject: Meet

Donna –
Anytime you are ready, we can meet and brainstorm about direction, logo design, brochure, fundraising ideas, etc. I am at your disposal.
Just let me know when you want to meet to get started.
Take care.
Cynthia Montello

I still didn't pick up the phone. I'm not sure why. Exhaustion. Fear of failure. A need for space. I don't know.

I didn't make the call.

"I'll rest through the holidays, concentrate on the kids, on healing, on getting my energy back. Then I'll call," I told myself.

Meanwhile, the folks who held my hand through it all seemed as happy as I was that the chemo was done.

To: donnahicken@firstcoastnews.com
Subject: 'from Donna's Journal'

Dear Donna.......... Congrats! You did it...no-mo-chem-o!!!!!! Yay, Yippeee, Yahooooo!!! I am so proud of you! All of us in the "Survivor Sisterhood" are proud of you,

181

and I know each and every one of us thank you from the bottoms of our hearts for letting us be a part of your life, your experience, your family.

You allowed us all to take a peak at a wonderful, brave woman. Now, perhaps, others may be more open and understanding to those of us that have "been there, done that." I consider it an honor and a privilege to have been able to follow your treatments and subsequent success! Keep up the good work, and know that God does have a plan for you, and He will reveal it in His timing.

God Bless you, bald head and all! Keep laughing and smiling!

Melissa Flowers

To: donnahicken@firstcoastnews.com
Subject: Hello

Hi, you don't know me from the man in the moon, but I must write to tell you I am so proud of you for your fantastic personality and fortitude. You set a marvelous example for other people who have some tough struggles in life and we all want you to enjoy a very happy and healthy life. thanx for just being you.

P J Panella (St. Augustine)

To: donnahicken@firstcoastnews.com
Subject: 'from Donna's Journal'

Dear Donna,

Thank you so much for being such an inspiration to me these past 6 months. I know that you letting us in on your most private thoughts has helped so many people who are struggling with their treatments. You give them hope that they too can make it through. You have helped me in a different way...

On October 23, 1998, my dear sister was killed in a fire in Ponte Vedra Beach. She left behind her then 9 year old daughter. My parents and my husband and I are raising her precious girl. Unfortunately, there has been no closure as her case remains open and unsolved. At times, I find it unbearable to live with. Then I see that life is difficult for so many people. God never promised it would be easy, he just promised he would carry us through the difficult times.

I am so happy that he has carried you through these last 6 months. My prayers for you are ones of total healing. You have made it through these difficult times, I know my family and I can as well. You represent hope, faith and so much courage.
Thanks again for keeping me going.
Love,
Angie Mohilowski

To: donnahicken@firstcoastnews.com
Subject: 'from Donna's Journal'

Hi Donna:
Thank you for making your Chemo public, and congratulations on getting through it. I bet not many people could do all that medication and still do your difficult job as professionally as you do it.

My wife Tish is 38, and the only time she'd go to a doctor was when she had the flu or something. We've moved all over the country and she's avoided having doctors ask her about checkups by changing doctors every time we moved. (I don't think she likes doctors.)

I've encouraged (begged) her to go for preventive checkups, but she dug her heels in... until a couple of nights passed when you weren't on the news, after saying you'd be going for Chemo. She said "Where's Donna tonight?" I didn't comment.

A couple of days later she was getting long-overdue checkups, and she was fine, and she says she'll be a regular now. Your example was a lot more persuasive than my words.

Thank you for being a great role model for my Tish-a-Poo.
Harvey Slentz

To: donnahicken@firstcoastnews.com
Subject: 'from Donna's Journal'

Hi Donna-
We are sooooooooooooooo happy for you that chemo is over!!! Remember us, Samantha is your San Jose Cath. buddy (8yr old)? Well, just a note from us to say we are so proud of you! You have had such courage and strength, and we can do all things through Him who strengthens us!!! When you talked about the plan God has for you, I think He already accomplished part of that plan to have you share your story with all of us, let us be there to encourage you, but also let you show us that with Him, and with family and friends and an awesome sense of humor, you did it! Our prayers for healing and strength

are being answered. I believe this so strongly, Donna. Keep the faith, and please keep us posted as your journal is so wonderful to read each week.

I had my last steroid injection for an ongoing back injury at Baptist today and (although minor in the grand scheme) makes me feel a month short of 140 instead of 40! I can relate to feeling ancient!!! So hearing you talk about God's plan refocused my thought process today to His plan for me instead of feeling sorry for myself!

Last time I wrote, I think I made you feel like you were not going through something as hard when I talked about losing our 3-month old son and I did not intend that!!!! I just think once we go through a life-altering event, we are all able to be more compassionate when we see others going through a difficult time. What I see is how strong and open you are and how you are doing things already for others facing breast cancer. It is the ripple effect — or more of that plan of His to be there for each other. And look how your words helped me today. So just wanted to say thanks for once again sharing your thoughts.
Love, Nancy Buckler

P.S. My 15-year-old Josh plays football at BK (your old stomping ground) and just got bumped up from JV to Varsity last week!! He is on cloud nine! Don't know if he'll play (he is 6"3" and 250 already as a sophomore !!!!) but he's happy to be in uniform on the sidelines for the last few games. Last home game will be this Thurs. nite @ BK against Episcopal. Then the playoffs... Samantha is not as enthused about MORE games to go to but we are proud of him! Go Crusaders!! We'll keep you posted... :)

To: NancyBuckler
Subject: RE: 'from Donna's Journal'

Hi Nancy!
You are too sweet! Thank you so much for all the support and the prayers. It's such a gift... and it makes me feel like anything is possible. I am so very glad to be through with chemo. Tell Samantha hi for me... and tell Josh I said "go big red!" Do they still say that at Kenny? They did when I was there... but that was a million years ago. I know you are proud! Anyway... thanks again for the kind words and the encouragement. It means the world. God bless you and your family,
Donna

To: donnahicken@firstcoastnews.com
Subject: 'from Donna's Journal'

Congratulations & Wahoo on your final treatment. I feel I know you as we spend every evening together & I too am a Jax native and BK alumni. I took care of my Mother thru her battle with cancer so I know how important prayers and support are. You are in mine daily. God bless you for your courage. You are in good hands and in my world you have WON!!!!.
Saundra Floyd

To: donnahicken@firstcoastnews.com
Subject: 'from Donna's Journal'

I am so happy for your latest rewards!!!! You are in my prayers. I hope things keep going well. Keep the faith and you will get stronger every day! Before too long, you

will be back to running marathons with your spikey blond
hair flowing in the breeze!!! :-)
Have a great day!
Chrisie Karpowicz

Day by day the alien was releasing its grip. My mind and my
body were starting to come into mutual focus as entities I
recognized. The haze was lifting.

Donna's Journal
Home > Health
November 11 , 2002

Hello Friends!

Well I must be feeling better. The evidence is
everywhere. I actually made it to the top of the stadium
to watch the Jaguars game on Sunday... then down for
all the junk food I could handle at half time... then back
up to scream myself hoarse in the second half. Goooooooo
Jags!

I can finally run...albeit slowly...and breathe at the
same time. My son has decided it's open season on
tackling mommy again. And the most convincing proof...
I forgot my hair today.
If I am going to be totally truthful...that has happened
before. Usually though, I remember by the time I get to
the car...or down the street. Today I made it all the way
in to work before I realized I had forgotten my hair at
home.

That can only mean one thing. My mind is finding better places to be. I am feeling better.

Thanks for caring and for all your wonderful messages of congratulation.

Talk to you soon. Have a great week and God bless!

Donna

My senses were coming alive. Sight, smell, taste, sound, touch. Tim was enjoying my rebirth.

"And where would you like to eat today?" he asked, relishing the question.

"I want to go to Sliders and eat oysters. I want oysters, and I want a Corona."

It was Saturday. Now weeks after the end of my chemotherapy. Food was good again. The metal plate gone from my mouth.

We hopped on our beach cruisers and pedaled north.

"Has the sky ever been this blue?" I asked.

"Never," Tim said smiling.

We guided our bikes to the rack in front of the restaurant and settled into one of the wooden tables on the outside patio.

"Hi there, it's great to see you two again. It's been awhile." The waitress barely got the words out of her mouth before I gave my order.

"We'll have two dozen raw please, and dos Corona's con limon por favor."

I was the man found on the deserted island, seeing real food for the first time in months.

"Are these the best oysters you have ever eaten?"

"Ever," Tim said.

I was busy stuffing oysters in my mouth, and the cracker wrappers under the basket in front of us when the idea came to me.

"I've got it!"

"Got what?"

"The invention that's going to make us rich?"

Tim rolled his eyes. He'd heard this about a million times before.

"We invent a receptacle for the cracker wrappers. Something with a retractable top. Then people can eat their oysters and the wrappers don't go flying all over the place."

"Oh, Phil might actually like that one," Tim said.

My 5:30 co-anchor Phil Amato and I have always dreamed of inventing something that would make us millions. Over the years we have come up with some doozies. Running tights with rip away Velcro was one of my personal favorites.

Phil is real. He is a man who knows there is life beyond television news. He doesn't define himself by it. He appreciates simple pleasures. Those things most of us take for granted. He takes his family to Disney almost every weekend, and still loves it. Every Friday he cooks a special meal at home and taunts us with the details on the set.

"Salmon on the plank tonight guys." His eyes light up as he's talking.

Plotting these crazy inventions with him was a delight. I couldn't wait to tell Phil about the plan.

"Hey Phillipee," I chimed as I swept past his cubicle at the office Monday afternoon.

"Hey Donna D. How's it going?"

I put my purse and make up on my desk and peered over the low wall that separates Phil's stuff from mine.

"Phil, I finally have the idea that's going to do it?"

"Yeah?"

Phil and I proceeded to draw out the "invention" and make a plan to get it patented. We always did this. We never followed through.

A month ago, I wouldn't have known or cared about any such far flung silliness, much less had the energy to plot with Phil over it.

189

"Good to see that spark back in your eye, Donna," Phil said.

Sure enough. As I stared in the mirror putting on my make-up before the show, there it was glistening back at me. Along with the faint outline of an eyebrow and a patch of sprouting lashes.

TWELVE

Taxi!

I stepped off the plane at Kennedy airport, pulling my hat down and my scarf up.

"Well girlfriend, here we are in the Big Apple," Andrea exclaimed.

Andrea always makes an announcement for posterity whenever we travel together.

Her sons, Christopher and Michael huddled beside her as we made our way through the terminal and out the other side where a sea of yellow cabs sat revving and ready to go.

"One, two, three, four, five, six…, geez… ten, 11."

"Drew! What ARE you doing?" I asked. "You've got to keep walking. It's freezing out here."

Danielle was holding my hand. Drew brought up the rear with my friend Nancy Saalfield who cares for the kids while I'm at work.

Drew's eyes were riveted on the waiting taxis.

"Mommy, Tim told me to count all the cabs I see and let him know how many."

"Wonderful. You should be up to about a zillion by the time we get to the hotel."

"Where's ours?" Drew asked.

"We aren't taking a cab today Drew-dog."

I scanned the parking lot looking for our car. There were too many of us for one cab, and besides I figured the kids would get a kick out of going first class.

There it is.

"We're going in that." I pointed to a stretch limo where a driver was holding a sign that said *Hicken*.

"That's my name," Drew said as if someone had just thrown magic dust on us all.

"Wow!" said Michael. "Cool."

Drew and Michael were 7 and 8 respectively. Chris 12 and Danielle 10. They got along beautifully.

"OK everybody, let's get a picture," Andrea instructed.

This was a trip Andrea and I had made many times. We spent 99 percent of our time shopping.

I was determined to bring the kids this year. I wanted them to see New York at Christmas.

More, I wanted them to see New York with ME at Christmas.

It was always something I resolved to do *next year*. No more.

"Never take another day for granted," I thought, still dreading my first post chemo tests.

It was late November, almost Thanksgiving. New York was wrapped up like a larger than life Christmas present. Enormous sparkling snowflakes were draped across busy streets. The toy soldiers in front of Radio City Music Hall were doing their holiday march. Giant bowls with boulder sized ornaments beckoned shoppers to stores.

"How will we live without shopping?" Andrea asked in mock dismay. "I'm having withdrawals already."

"Oh honey, we'll be so busy ice skating in Rockefeller Plaza we won't even miss it."

Andrea leaned over throwing me a bewildered look. For all the times we had been here we had never once done the mandatory tourist drill.

Nancy and Drew were already plotting their first ice-skating adventure while Danielle and Christopher seemed intent on pushing every button in the limo. Michael's mouth was wide open as he stared at the endless line of skyscrapers that blocked the sun.

"I haven't been back here since 9-11," I whispered to Andrea as the limo snaked its way through the streets of Manhattan.

"It must have been so different," she said.

I had come to New York a few weeks after 9-11. The first week of October 2001. We had a lot of local relief people who were helping out and the station sent me up to follow them around.

Jon Frankel offered me a place to stay. A photographer from one of our sister stations in New York met me to shoot our stories.

Jon and I sat up half the night talking about what had happened. Each of us dipping spoons into our own half gallon cartons of Starbucks Coffee Ice Cream.

New York was Jon's home, and this had seemed even more surreal to him than to most.

"I found myself taking a lot of pictures," he said.

Jon is a journalist by profession. Photography is a passion.

His images of candlelight vigils and aimless faces spoke volumes.

"People were lost, just wandering," he said. " Everyone was looking for someone. There were lists up everywhere with names."

The next day as my photographer and I navigated the city, that part of the story had mostly given way to the recovery effort. Lower Manhattan was covered in a thick gray dust.

One restaurant owner kept his place open at all hours, serving the workers, police, firefighters and volunteers for free.

"It's a nice thing you're doing," I said, camera rolling.

"It's NOT nice," he said in his thick New York accent "It's the right thing to do."

People still gathered to mourn, some holding precious memories of those lost.

Others prayed. Some cried. Many left messages of sorrow or support scrawled on signs in any available space. The gaping hole in the skyline was almost unfathomable. The pall of grief over this city as palpable as the lump had been in my breast.

"It was very different." I said to Andrea. "Very sad. It's good to see New York is back."

"Can we go to Ground Zero?" Christopher asked.

It's amazing how kids can't seem to hear you when you've barked at them for the fifth time to dress for school, but whisper something you don't wish to share, and they've got every word down to the syllable.

"Yes, Chris, at some point," Andrea said.

We had planned all along to take the kids to Ground Zero. It was a history lesson in living color. But I wasn't looking forward to it.

"What do you guys want to do first?" I asked.

We had several hours before we were scheduled to see *The Lion King* on Broadway.

"ICE SKATING," they all screamed in unison.

Nancy smiled. Andrea shrugged.

I was a bald girl in a hat with one mission only. Make this the trip of my life with my kids.

"Sounds great to me," I said. "Let's check in at the hotel and go for it."

The day was bitter cold. The following week I would be in Costa Rica with Tim. I couldn't imagine feeling warm.

"Mom, look at me, watch this," Drew screamed as he hurled his body around the skating rink.

Drew had been on the ice for all of five minutes and he was already soaked from falling. He skated as fast and hard as he could until he lost his balance, and then just went flying, feet up in the air and onto his bottom.

Danielle, meanwhile, maintained a death grip on the railing so tight that her knuckles were blue.

"Danielle sweetie, believe me, if Mom can do this, so can you. Why don't you hold my hand and we'll go together."

"No Mom, I'm fine right here, thanks."

She eventually let go and made her way tentatively around the rink with me. Every now and then Drew would zoom by, nearly knocking us both from our feet.

Three hours later we collapsed on our beds at the hotel and tried to recharge for the evening.

I had already asked more of my body in one day than I had in six months, but this kind of exhaustion felt good.

That night as we crossed Times Square to the theatre, I found myself staring at my children. The light in their eyes was brighter than the spectacle before us. A new world was opening in front of them and I was there watching it open.

"Why are you crying Mommy?" Danielle grabbed my hand.

"Just feeling grateful, baby doll."

Grateful doesn't really begin to cover it. For the second time I had faced the prospect of death, only to be given new life. I felt more deeply. Colors were more vibrant. I was aware of every breath. Nothing seemed insignificant. A great gift in a way. The kind I would have never wished to receive, but now found myself embracing.

Drew tugged on my shirt.

"Mommy, can I have a bag of gummy worms for the show?"

Drew finds it virtually impossible to sit for any length of time without food.

"Yes Drew, but share."

"Moooooooom."

I can only tell you that the part of *The Lion King* I actually stayed awake for that night was phenomenal. Watching my children watch was more breath-taking than the costumes.

The next day we started at the crack of dawn. A bone-chilling wind swept the waterfront at Battery Park. We gazed at the Statue of Liberty, then began the trek to Ground Zero.

The scene could not have been more removed from the one I remembered.

Tall chain-link fences flanked the footprints of the twin towers. It was clean, antiseptic. Tourists were chatting and taking pictures like you would at the zoo.

"Can you hold me up so I can see?" Drew asked.

I did my best.

"I don't really see anything," he said.

There isn't much there anymore Drew, except for where the

towers used to be.

"But there are people down there, right?" Christopher was looking hard at the ground.

"Yes, a lot of people," Andrea said solemnly.

Like the other tourists, we snapped some pictures to mark the moment and we headed back uptown.

Tragedies happen and life goes on.

The thought of my own mortality swept over me.

Life is for the living as it should be I suppose.

The rest of the day we packed in more of New York than I had seen in a half a dozen trips.

From the Rockettes to the Empire State Building. In the subway we heard a symphony made entirely of pots and pans. And of course we had to return to exhaust ourselves one final time at the ice rink in Rockefeller Plaza.

The next morning before we left, I even managed a slow but satisfying sunrise run in Central Park. An act that even in healthier days I never once took for granted.

We could have been there for five weeks, or for five minutes.

"Wave goodbye to New York, kids," Andrea instructed, the city now shrinking from the window of the plane.

"So how many cabs did you count Drew?"

"I don't know," he said, shaking his head. "I stopped counting around 799."

THIRTEEN

¡Con Mucho Gusto!

Donna's Journal
Home > Health
November 28, 2002

I hope you had a wonderful Thanksgiving. I sure did. In addition to absolutely stuffing myself at my aunt and uncle's house, I just feel that I have so much to be thankful for.

From big things like... well... being alive, to small things like watching my daughter fly a kite on the beach, life is good.

My hair is starting to come back in slowly but surely. My daughter calls me the fuzz ball...but hey it's something. I am heading out of town for a vacation/ celebration for the next two weeks so don't worry when you see I'm not here... I'm just relaxing and having fun.

I hope to come back looking a little less tired. Even though my chemo is done... it's going to take a while before my body gets back to full speed... but I'm feeling better all the time.

Yes there is much to be thankful for...and I certainly count all of you among my many blessings.

Have a great TWO weeks... and God bless.

Donna

"OK, what's our strategy this time?" I gave Tim a conspiratorial smile.

We were trying to figure out how to beat our friends Louis and Carrie at spades. Well, Louis' own special version of the card game anyway.

"I'm not sure it's possible," Tim said. "You just finished chemo and I'm a real blonde, so I don't know if we have what it takes."

Louis and Carrie own a little piece of paradise in Northern Costa Rica. We discovered it just after our engagement, and make as many trips as our vacation schedules will allow.

This time, we were going to be there for two glorious weeks. While the folks at home were enduring the most consistent cold in eons, we would be swimming and surfing in clear 80 degree waters with eternally blue skies, warm tropical breezes and temperatures near 90. I couldn't think of a better way to rejuvenate.

We left Jacksonville bundled up like Eskimos, but stripped down to shorts in the Atlanta airport before boarding the plane to Costa Rica.

Once on the ground, an hour's drive on bumpy dirt roads took us to our destination.

"Hola Donna, Hola Timatao!" Sandra was coming toward us with her arms spread wide.

Sandra is a fixture at Louis and Carrie's place. She's five feet of warm, friendly Costa Rican hospitality. Her caramel colored skin and dark brown eyes are outdone only by her broad smile. There is something mischievous in her expression and something very genuine.

Hospitality is not at all hard to find in this Central American country. But Sandra takes it to another level. Over the past couple of years she has become a friend, despite our inability to learn Spanish.

We usually arrive with a handful of useful words in tow. We can say "Hello, how are you?" (*Hola, Como esta?*) To which the

198

answer usually comes *Bien, usted?* (Fine, and you?) We can ask for a bottle of water *botilla de agua*; or a beer, *cervasa*. We can say "thank you" (*gracias*), and we can sometimes fit in the occasional menu item or surf question.

Each time, by the day we leave we have added a half dozen words to our repertoire, courtesy of Sandra.

Each time, we forget them before we step foot back in the United States.

It's pathetic really. But what with me just finishing chemo and Tim being a real blonde and all, I didn't see that changing much this time.

Sandra seems to enjoy the challenge. At the very least she is kind enough not to call us idiots to our faces.

"Your room is ready," Sandra said still appraising our appearances.

Sandra gave me an extra squeeze.

"You feeling better?"

"I am now," I said.

Sandra made a running motion with her arms.

"You running?"

"Si, running," I smiled.

Sandra nodded. I get the feeling she thinks I run a little too much, although she has never said it.

"What do you say we go unpack all our bags?" I said, turning to Tim.

"Sounds bien, see you soon, Sandra."

The best thing about traveling to Costa Rica is the packing. There is none. We each bring a backpack with a few pairs of shorts and a few bathing suits, a book, a toothbrush and toothpaste. That's all.

Tim brought his surfboard down the first time and after an emotional goodbye to his "buddy" he left it there.

That's how sure we were that this place would be our second home. The first time we made the trip, we sat at our favorite table, gazing at the sun as it seared it's way into the deepening sky. We had both been instantly enchanted the first day.

"If we still feel as good on Sunday about this place as we do today," Tim said, "we'll go ahead and book another trip."

Needless to say, we did, and Tim's board stayed.

It's always waiting for him in our room when we return. My surfing, if you could call it that, is such that I can fall off just about any board they have lying around, and I generally do.

There is no luxury where we are. Nothing most people would consider luxurious anyway. We have hot water, tasty food, and a room with a panoramic view of the ocean. Everything we need. Nothing we don't.

There are enormous lizards everywhere. One of the creatures sits on top of a Mexican tile roof next to the open air restaurant on the second floor. Louis calls him the answer lizard because his head is constantly bobbing up and down.

"Ask him anything you like," Louis says. "He'll always say yes."

Louis is a character like no other. He moved here from St. Augustine in the early 70's. He is responsible for making this area a sea turtle preserve. Most of the people he hires used to make their living harvesting turtle eggs and selling them. Now they are part of the cause.

Louis is a gracious host, and an avid surfer. He's funny and serious, and I still have absolutely no idea when he's trying to be either.

Carrie is much younger. Tall with long blonde hair, she is smart as a whip and shy around most people. She writes beautifully and has a head for business. I could describe both of them as somewhat eccentric, although the older I get I wonder which one of us isn't.

"Hi kids," Louis waved as we headed down the stairs on our way to the beach.

"How's life in the real world? How are the dual dopplers?"

There are no televisions at Louis' place, and only one phone at the front desk which rarely works. Louis keeps up though. He always seems to know more about what's going on at home than we do.

"How are you, and Carrie?" I asked reaching up to give him a hug.

"Raring to beat you two at spades," he said.

"Come on. Don't you two need a new challenge? We have hardly proven ourselves worthy," Tim said.

"Oh you'll win this time," Louis said laughing.

He looked at Tim, who was standing there with his surfboard tucked under his arm.

"The sea breeze is already in today, but we've got a good swell coming."

Louis was well aware he was telling Tim something he already knew.

"I'm still gonna' get wet," Tim said.

"Of course, have fun."

Louis and Tim understand each other. They both have a love for the ocean, and while the perfect wave would be welcome, it's all good.

Invariably some young surfer dude will walk in complaining about how bad the waves are and Tim and Louis will just look at each other and smile.

I trailed Tim down to the ocean, sporting a baseball cap to cover my now fuzzy head. The warmth of the afternoon sun covered the beach like a blanket. I let it swaddle my skin, and comfort my bones. I couldn't imagine feeling cold.

"It says something about me," I told Tim as he joined me on the beach after testing the water.

"When I was in New York, freezing, I couldn't imagine this kind of warmth. I mean really couldn't get myself there. Here, the exact opposite. I'm like that with sunny and cloudy days too. Maybe that's why I got myself so mired in the chemo. So sure it was never going to be OK. I just couldn't see around it."

"Sounds human," Tim said.

There wasn't a day I woke up that I didn't think first about the cancer, but it was starting to seem more like a distant dream than my worst nightmare. The POW was beginning to sense freedom, still on guard, but allowing my overworked mind some rest.

I was grateful that Louis didn't bring up the cancer. No one did really, except for that first vague inquiry from Sandra. They knew I was here to leave it behind, to heal, to find my way back.

I knew when I returned I'd be facing those first critical tests. It was there nagging in the back of my brain, but only in the back. I didn't let it go further than that.

"How about if we take a long walk on the beach, take a shower and then head to Kike's for some pool?" Tim said.

"Are you already trying to schedule my day?" I chided.

Tim is a schedule freak. He literally schedules his day down to the minute. Each morning he pulls out a white legal pad and charts his course. I have it memorized. Surely he must too, but he still does it, every day.

5:35 up
6:00 radio weather
7:10 radio weather
7:15 run
8:00 radio weather
8:30 Mass
9:30 run with Donna/Surf
11:00 lunch
12:00 siesta
1:35 shower
2:00 leave for work

It goes on from there until we get off the air at 11:35 p.m. Then the next day he starts again.

"No schedules, just a suggestion," he said throwing his hands back in the air.

"Perfect."

The short walk to Kike's (pronounced Key-Kays) is down another dusty road, flanked by trees and fields and the occasional howler monkey. The first time I ever heard a howler monkey it became evident how they got their names. I cannot imagine how such a blood-curdling sound could ever come from something so small. It's sort of a cross between the Hound of the Baskervilles and a banshee. Hideous.

Kike's Place is down a small hill. A little hole-in-the-wall with a grass roof and a long wooden bar. It also houses the only pool table within walking distance.

Kike is a happy man. He looks to be in his 70's, always shirtless and always smiling. Always.

On Tuesdays Kike has Karoke night. Of course it's in Spanish so we don't understand a word, but it's fun to watch.

This is where Tim and I hold the international pool championships.

I win more than he does, but it's usually on a technicality.

He can run the table, be poised for victory, and then the white ball follows the eight ball into the hole. He scratches.

Tonight would be no exception.

"Victory is mine, Timatao," I teased as the cue ball betrayed him again.

Tim stared at the corner pocket in disbelief, and dropped his head.

"Please tell me you are not surprised," I said.

"I can't believe I keep doing that."

"You've heard, of course, the definition of insanity," I said. "You keep doing the same thing over and over again, expecting a different outcome."

"I need a cervasa." Tim motioned to the waitress with his empty bottle.

"Imperial, por favor."

The night sky was black and bursting with stars as we walked hand in hand back to the hotel. The scene made me feel incredibly grateful.

"Life is good," I said.

"Yes it is."

The next two weeks were filled with old pleasures and new ones. Our friends Nanci and Jerre Weckhorst were there. We usually try to make our trips coincide. They make the trek from coastal South Carolina.

Nanci is a former East Coast Surfing Champion. She has an incredibly long blondish gray pony tail and compassionate blue eyes. She makes sails for boats and still surfs like a pro. Jerre walks like he's in a brace, but in the water he can still move. He rides a long red and white board with small handles he's attached to the sides. In his book the waves are NEVER good enough, except of course for one incredibly good wave that Jerre never tires of describing. He and a group including long time Jacksonville surfing guru Roger Wood paddled out years ago on a day that surfers would call epic.

A little too epic for Jerre.

"I didn't want the wave, but I didn't have a choice. I could try to ride it in, or let it crush me. I'm telling you, you could've driven a semi through that tube. I probably rode it for a half a mile."

We have heard that story at least six times, and it's still fun to listen to Jerre tell it. The neat thing is, you can watch Nanci, who has probably heard it about 3000 times, and she's right there, hanging on every word.

She and Jerre have been together since they were kids, and they still have that youthful shine for each other. Carrie says they pick the same room every time they come because they like the way the bed squeaks. Both are a joy to be around.

We also met a new couple from California. She is an interior designer. We spent much of the second week talking about sofa colors. I was trying to pick one out. She laughed when I finally raced down to the pool one day with a long strip of papaya I snatched from Tim's lunch plate.

"This is it!" I said, unfolding a napkin to reveal my choice.

"Well there's a new one," she said. "Never once have I had a client give me a piece of fruit as a color choice."

She ended up sending some swatches to the house when we

got home. I eventually went with another color altogether.

Mostly we surfed, and read, and lazed around in the hammocks that surround the property.

And we ran.

"We are so fortunate to be able to do all this," I said to Tim as we loped down the beach one morning.

"It sounds like there's a 'but' in there someplace."

"But there are so many people who can't."

Tim knew what was coming.

"I have got to get myself focused on this foundation when we get home. God has been urging me on to this for so long and I keep putting it off."

"You needed time to regroup, Donna."

"I know but it's not quiet voices anymore. God is whispering in my ear like a freight train these days. There are women who can't afford their basic treatments, women who can't afford to pay their bills while they try to get through this horrible disease. They wouldn't even begin to dream about recovering in a tropical paradise. They just want to pay the electric bill."

"OK, I hear you. Why don't you touch base with Steve Prom when we get home and really get this thing moving."

Steve Prom is a friend. He is also a well-respected attorney who has done a lot of foundation work. He and I had already been through the paperwork to set up the foundation, but I had let it go for months.

When we said our good-byes to Costa Rica, having lost yet again to Louis and Carrie in spades, I headed home with a purpose.

"So do you think I can really make this foundation work?" I asked Tim on the plane.

"Well, you did just finish chemo…"

"…but I'M not a real blonde," I interrupted.

"Well, there you go," he said. "Chemo wears off. You'll do just fine."

FOURTEEN

Hallelujah, Hair She Comes

"Steve Prom, please." I pressed the receiver to my ear, anxious for Steve to pick up. Ten seconds later his secretary came to the phone.

"I'm sorry, Steve is out of the office for the holidays, would you like to leave a message?"

"No thanks, I'll call back."

It was my first day back in the office after Costa Rica. I hung up the phone and stared at my computer. *Do I dare log on?*

I was anxious to check my e-mail, but at the same time dreading what I might see. *If I look now, I'll never get my newscast done. First things first.*

I clicked the icon that takes me to the rundown for the day's broadcasts and began reviewing and revising the stories I would deliver in the 5:30p.m. show.

When I got my first job in news back in 1984, I did a lot more writing for the daily shows. In fact, I was it. I was the morning anchor and I reported for the evening shows. I would come in at 4 a.m., produce my short newscasts, write them, edit them on tape and anchor them. Then I'd set up my interviews, rush out with a photographer at 9 a.m. and spend the rest of the day chasing stories. I would usually get home about 7 p.m. Just in time to eat dinner, go to bed and start all over. I actually had it good. I had some friends in other television markets who also had to shoot their own video and run their own teleprompter with a foot pad from under the desk!

The problem is, when you are a control freak, you don't like to give up sovereignty on anything.

When I first came to Jacksonville as a weekend anchor in 1988, I insisted on writing the entire newscast. That didn't always play well with producers who felt that I was taking away the one thing they loved to do.

"But they are my words. I have to say them my way," I would argue.

Plus writing was always my favorite part of the job, the reason I entered journalism in the first place.

The producer who finally broke me was a woman named Cathy MacFeaters. We began working together just before my transition to the Monday through Friday evening broadcasts.

Cathy is a talented writer. I say this because I virtually could not distinguish the copy she wrote from my own.

"If I'm a good producer," she said, "I learn your style, the way you talk and write, and I can write in that style for you."

"OK," I relented. "Tell you what. I'll start writing at the top of the newscast and go down, you start at the bottom and go up and we'll meet in the middle."

"Deal."

I loved working with Cathy. We were one mind working in two people when it came to news writing and most especially news judgement.

She later went on to become a news director at the Gannett affiliate in Austin, Texas.

Cathy always had a low tolerance for B.S. It was one of the things I respected most about her. In the end, the politics of the news business got to her. All the noise that can drown out the pure love of chasing the truth, the turn of an enlightened phrase, the satisfaction of tying it all together in a neat little bow, on deadline. That noise just became too loud.

She got out. Journalism's loss.

These days, while the anchors have input, the producers make the decisions on what goes into the shows, and they usually write the lion's share of the broadcast.

Like most anchors, I still write some, change things around to suit my style, correct grammar mistakes, and of course complain that those 20 something year-old producers just don't know their stuff "like we did."

My 11 p.m. co-anchor Alan Gionet and I laugh about it sometimes.

"Why don't they at least realize we've learned a few things over the years that might help them?" he asks.

"Because it's part of being 22 to think you know everything."

"And I suppose it's part of being 42 to think when you're 22 you know nothing?"

"Exactly."

Actually, our producers are great about asking questions and most seem to want to learn. It's not their fault that most don't remember a U.S. president before Bill Clinton.

I cleaned up the last bit of copy, and headed for "the office."

Our front desk secretary Bonita was standing in the ladies restroom.

"Girl, I am so tired of taking calls about you," she said, throwing her arms in the air. "People are worried something's wrong because you've been gone for two weeks."

"I'm afraid to open my e-mail," I said.

"Well open it, and get started, maybe I can get some rest."

Bonita smiled, but I knew that it was always an ordeal for anyone who had to answer the phones when I disappeared for a while. Even if I was gone for one day, people often feared the worst.

I waited until after the newscast to log on to my messages from "Donna's Journal."

To: donnahicken@firstcoastnews.com
Subject: Merry Christmas

Donna... please keep smiling... I am still praying... I am

sure the angel helped you a lot. Man I was worried about you not being on TV this past few days... so I went to Donna's journal and thank goodness you are on a vacation. You need a rest I am sure but we miss your smiling face and of course your laughter. We are so proud of you.
Have a Merry Christmas and may 2003 bring the best of everything for you and your family.
In Friendship and love
Colleen Davison

To: donnahicken@firstcoastnews.com
Subject: days off

Donna,
I hope you enjoyed your days off. I was worrying about you until I came across your journal... That's a nice thing for us fans & keeps us up to date a bit. We don't want to be a pain but, we care about you and pray for you.
I had a bout with Melanoma but, I was fortunate that it was only growing superficial. I always live with a fear of it coming back. If it gets to your brain, heart or your lungs it will kill you. And, it's a shame that people have to feel less attractive without a beautiful golden tan ... :o(
I try not to let it bother me. I'm alive. You're a beautiful lady wig, or no wig. I'm glad you're having fun with that. Shoot, I'd be trying out all kinds of different dos.... :o)
I just look forward to your chipper & cheerful newscast every night.
be strong & believe,
Debra Hoffkins

To: Debra
Subject: RE: days off

Hi Debra,
My days off were awesome ... thanks. I didn't wear the wig one time!!! I really appreciate your words of encouragement. If I seem chipper... you have certainly helped make me that way. God bless and again...thanks for taking the time to write.
Donna

Time for an update.

Donna's Journal
Home > Health
December 16 , 2002

Hi folks!

Well it's sure good to be home! I had a fabulous vacation. Lots of sun and lots of sleep! I feel refreshed and ready to roll. I'm sure that will last until I hit the entrance to the mall to go Christmas shopping!! Here we are... just a week or so left... and I'm just starting. Oh well... you know me... I work best under deadlines. Don't give me too much time to do anything or it won't get done. Tell me I have five minutes to do it... I'm golden.

It was great to hear from all of you who e-mailed in to say hi or to give me an update or to make sure I was OK I appreciate you so much.

By the way...the hair is growing. I have a nice little short do working under the blonde locks. Hopefully

"Jennifer" and "Brenda" won't mind retiring in the near future. I hope "the girls" won't take it personally, but I can't wait!

Have a wonderful holiday season and keep in touch.

God bless,
Donna

The idea was starting to grow on me just like the hair under my wig.

My fuzz was getting thicker every day. In fact, in the past week or so it had graduated from fuzz to what I'd call baby duck hair. Brenda and Jennifer had been good to me, but I was getting impatient for a change.

Three weeks later, with all the Christmas shopping over and the New Year beginning, I finally got up the nerve to ask my boss. Sort of.

"Hey Mike, I've got a question for you."

"What's up?"

"I'm going to take off my wig today."

"How is that a question?"

"What do you mean?"

"I mean that's not a question, it's a statement."

"OK then, thanks."

I may be one of the only people in the world who can render Mike McCormick speechless. It wasn't that I expected an argument from Mike, I just couldn't risk it.

As insurance I left "Jennifer" in the drawer at home.

That night the girl with the baby duck hair delivered the news. The response was incredible. I came to the conclusion that it wouldn't have mattered if I'd gone on the air with a purple mohawk, people wanted to make me feel good again, and they did.

To: donnahicken@firstcoastnews.com
Subject: 'from Donna's Journal'

Donna -
I just wanted to take a minute to tell you how GREAT you look with the short new do. I am sure that "Jennifer" and "Brenda" don't mind being retired. You just look so wonderful and I hope that you are feeling equally as wonderful.
Angie Judah

To: donnahicken@firstcoastnews.com
Subject: (none)

Donna,

Congratulations that you are back into your own hair again. You look wonderful!!

Donna, I don't think you realize the magnitude of your impact in our area with regard to cancer. I am an academic dean at a college that specializes in training individuals in medicine disciplines. I never broach the subject of cancer without your name surfacing. Most importantly, with the mention of your name, I see hope in the eyes of those who are talking about that dreaded "C" word. Many of them know someone who is fighting a battle, many of whom are struggling in their fight. They somehow conclude that if Donna is OK, their loved one will be also.

You are a member of an elite segment of society: those who are survivors. You exemplify each day what all of us survivors come to know: There is Life After Cancer!!

213

I want you to know how very grateful I am for your continued courage. As you continue to live a wonderful life (one that happens also to include cancer), may all those who are struck with our dreaded disease come to learn what you display each day: that there is hope. May God return unto you blessings in abundance for your work and labor of love.
Your fellow survivor,
Reba Hoffman

To: donnahicken@firstcoastnews.com
Subject: (none)

Happy New Year, Donna! May this be THE ONE...lots of love, happiness, and restored health.
You are still on our prayer list at St. John's Cathedral. Shall you stay in our active prayer list, or are you ready to go back to "no training wheels"? I bet you don't really miss Brenda. She certainly served you well!
So happy to see your own "crew cut."
All my best wishes. God bless!
Madge Bruner Hazen

To: Madge....
Subject: Thank you

Oh Gosh Madge....If my training wheels are your prayers I don't ever want to take them off! Thank you so much for the continued support...especially the prayers.
God bless.
Donna

To: donnahicken@firstcoastnews.com
Subject: keep it up!

Hi Donna
I was just about to send you an e-mail to tell you how beautiful you look with your "new" hair when my husband, Tony, came in to the room and said "Look at Donna, she looks just like a model." Keep up the good work. We are so glad you are doing so well.
Pat Braden

To: donnahicken@firstcoastnews.com
Subject: (no subject)

Glad to have your classic look back - you look GREAT !!!
Way to go TUFF STUFF !!!!!!!!!
George and Diane Harrison

To: donnahicken@firstcoastnews.com
Subject: 'from Donna's Journal'

I am a 53 year old grandmother so I'm not a pervert! I think you look beautiful with the short hair. You look so much healthier. Good luck to you and my prayers will still be with you.
Diane Millwood (Waycross, GA)

To: donnahicken@firstcoastnews.com
Subject: 'from Donna's Journal'

hey there—
saw you last night on the news—you look mah-va-lus!!!
great new make-up too — you go girl!!!!
Christine Holleman

To: Christine
Subject: RE: 'from Donna's Journal'

Thanks for the nice words. Feels good to have to wig off!
I appreciate the compliment on the make-up...believe it
or not though...same old stuff... I just have more color
without the lovely chemo.
Donna

To: donnahicken@firstcoastnews.com
Subject: Hair!

Wow! Donna, I am sooooo glad to see your hair again...
You are a very beautiful lady (inside as well as outside)
and I'm so glad to see your face "opened up" again... all
fresh and shining! You look mah-ve-lous! I have enjoyed
reading your journal and watching you on the news... I
have worried about you when you weren't on the set and
nothing was mentioned about you that day... I've been a
little out of "it" at times... was diagnosed with Hepatitis A
in 5/98 and take a lot of meds... actually, much less than
originally... it's my form of "chemotherapy"... only mine
just puts weight on me! I am now 55 and the grandmother
of twins... Jake and Grace. I KNOW why my Lord has
kept me alive since then... I am on disability now... have
autoimmune hepatitis with liver failure... the illnesses and
medications have caused some problems in my life... but
reading your journal has really helped me! I pray for you
and hope your "new" marriage is blessed!
In God's Love,

Cheryl Philips
Green Cove Springs

To: donnahicken@firstcoastnews.com
Subject: 'from Donna's Journal'

Hi,
Love your own hair. You look great with it short and you're lucky that you have the type of face to wear that style. Long hair is not for you. I am thrilled to see you look so look, your color is great and your eyes just shine. Thank God you're back to your old self. I pray you will never hear the C word again.
My daughter had thyroid cancer at the age of 25 and now 11 years later she is just fine. Her being a only child just about killed us but she was so brave and with a lot of prayer all went well.
May God bless you and your family with all good and great things. You seem like family, as you're in our home every night.
See you on TV, Pat Collins

To: donnahicken@firstcoastnews.com
Subject: 'from Donna's Journal'

Dear Donna,
Brief note to tell you how simply beautiful you are. Although I "adapted" to the girls, I just couldn't believe how gorgeous you are with your natural hair. Bless God, I have good health but should I ever be ill, I will always remember your courage, dignity and class. Thank you for the important lesson you have taught us all.
Continue with your progress as we all cheer you on.
Forever a fan,
Toi Wassing

P.S. Nosey question—what about the ring??? :)

217

To: donnahicken@firstcoastnews.com
Subject: YOU LOOK BEAUTIFUL

Hi Donna, I look forward to seeing you on the news, and last night, I couldn't stop saying to the Mrs., how great you look with you own hair. And how brave you are and what an inspiration you are to women and men. Hope you have a happy & healthy new year
One of your fans,
Louis Mastellone

To: donnahicken@firstcoastnews.com
Subject: You Look Great!

Donna. . . Donna. . . Donna!
Today I turned on the news and there you were with that gorgeous hairdo. I am so proud of you to have had the faith and courage to "hang in there" through all the things you have been through. Today you looked like the picture of health. I love the short hair cut and I hope you never have to go back to the wig again. All I can say is. . . YOU GO GIRL!
Good luck on everything the future holds for you.
Erma Battle

Donna's Journal
Home > Health
January 22, 2003

Hi folks!

I'm feeling a bit light-headed. I'm not sure whether it's from taking that load off my head... or all the beautiful phone calls... e-mails and letters I have received from you! Probably a bit of both. I've said it so many times... I can't believe how awesome you all are.

I felt a bit self-conscious the first day without "the girls" and you all made me feel so comfortable. If I live to be a hundred (and that's what I'm aiming for) I will never be able to thank you enough for your kindness and generosity. I have to admit...I feel much more myself now I can move my head... and know... for certain... that my hair will be moving with me and more importantly... in the same direction!

I have been taking a bit of time to vacation just to enjoy feeling good again and to build some strength back. I'm getting there. I must report though... that my son can still beat me at wrestling. He keeps getting bigger and I keep getting older. But hey... I can live with that. I just thank God for the "live" part.

Have a great weekend and keep in touch.

God bless you all,

Donna

Living was the bottom line after all. And I really was living again. So much so, that it worried me. My mind flashed back to that day at Mayo and the PET scan that threw my life into chaos for the second time.

Too happy, must be time for something bad to happen.

I pushed the thought to its hiding place in the back of my mind.

No time for that, I have too much to do.

My eyes slid to the date circled on the calendar at my desk.

January 31st – blood work.

219

FIFTEEN

Stress Test

Three months to the day after my last chemo treatment I walked into the Mayo Clinic to have my blood drawn. The day before I had done what I always do, tried to find reasons to cancel.

"I had to take something for a headache two days ago, what if that skews my numbers?"

"I'm just about to start my period. Maybe I should wait?"

"I'm just so slammed at work right now, I could put it off to next week."

Tim had heard every lame excuse in the book.

"Won't you just feel better when it's over?"

"That depends."

"Donna, I know you're nervous, but just think about how great it will feel to get some good news."

"Or how horrible it will feel to get some bad news."

"Do you want me to go with you?"

"It's a 30 second blood test."

"I can't win here can I?"

"Absolutely not."

In the end, I couldn't find an excuse that even approached acceptable, so I went.

Alone.

I was just too agitated to be around anyone else, even Tim.

As I entered the huge double glass doors from the parking lot, I felt that familiar wave of nausea.

Just get in and get out.

Val was waiting for me on the eighth floor.

"Hello girl, it's so great to see you."

Once again I was swept up in Val's bear hug.

"Good to see you too," I said, managing a weak smile.

"It's going to be fine, let's get this over with," she said, reading my mind.

If all went well, this would be my last trip to the eighth floor for blood work.

The rule for taking out a port-o-cath is wait until after the first tests. Good results and the third boob comes out, not good and it stays in. Once the port was out, I'd be relegated to the lab on the first floor, where the nurses draw lots, to see who has to try to stick the veinless one.

Val started toward me with the needle.

"Hey, don't forget my freezy spray," I said.

"Sorry."

Val grabbed the numbing spray and gave my port a good dousing.

"OK, deep breath... and we're in."

I watched the blood leave my body and enter the first of two large tubes.

Please be good to me. Don't betray me, please.

It's a wild thought, this worry that my own body could turn on me. I was willing the blood to make my life whole again.

Three excruciating days later, I was out shopping when I saw Edith's name flashing on my cell phone. I almost didn't answer.

I'll just let her leave a message and I'll call her back when I'm at home.

But the curiosity was too great.

"Hello Edith."

"How did you know it was me?"

"Magic."

"Are you sitting down?"

"No, I'm shopping, this would be an odd place to sit."

But I had already heard the tone of her voice. Edith would not toy with me if the news was bad.

"Great news, Donna. Your numbers are excellent."

Excellent!

"Even the marker?"

"Especially the marker. Best ever. Completely normal, 34."

I could see Edith's smile through the phone.

"Thank God," I said, realizing I hadn't taken a breath through the entire conversation.

I was so elated, I didn't want to ask the next question. Edith had planned a follow up PET scan right after my blood work.

"What about the PET scan? Are we still doing that?"

"No, I don't see a need for it right now. Maybe we will do one at some point just as a baseline, but these numbers are great. We'll just keep watching."

"Sounds like you are a bit surprised."

"Not surprised, but I didn't know. We have never done this marker test on you before you had cancer. We don't know what normal is for you. Not that I'm basing everything on that. Your other blood work is perfect. You know I don't like this marker test to begin with."

Edith began to launch into her well-documented feelings about the marker and its unpredictability, but I was no longer listening.

I'm NORMAL, and no PET scan. WAHOO!

I dropped what I was doing, ran to the car and called Tim, Mom, Julie, Andrea, my Aunt and Uncle, and basically everyone I'd ever known. The kids were still in school, and I had to fight the urge to run over and tell them. But that would have placed more importance on the test than I had ever wanted them to see.

I was also anxious to get to work and tell the viewers.

First, I made a bee-line to Mike's office.

"Got a second, boss?"

"You know, I always hate it when you say that because it usually means either you're mad at me, or you're going to be mad at me."

"No, I'm not mad. I just thought you should know that you are going to have to put up with me a little longer."

"Really?" Mike's face spread into a smile.

"Yep, tests were great. Completely normal. So looks like I'll live to be mad at you another day."

"Excellent."

I left Mike's office and went straight to my computer.

Donna's Journal
Home > Health
February 3, 2003

Hello Friends!

I was standing in Target today looking for school supplies and Valentines cards...and my cell phone rang. It was my doctor and she asked if I was sitting down. I assured her that this would not really be a good place to sit down...and instead held my breath. She was calling with the results of my first full post treatment work-up. The news was WONDERFUL!

For someone who likes to occasionally be different... just for the sake of being different... I have never been so happy to be called NORMAL in my whole life. I know it sounds dramatic... but the truth is...it is dramatic. Anyone who has been through cancer treatment will tell you that the long months of chemotherapy tend to work on one's confidence.

It's easy to be convinced by an exhausted body and mind that things will never be right again. Beyond that...just when the normalcy returns to life...it's time for that BIG checkup. I could get nauseated just walking into that clinic. Sweaty palms the whole bit. So to say that today's phone call was a huge relief would be the understatement of the century. It's the answer to so many prayers. Prayers that you have prayed with me. I couldn't wait to share the news with you. You've stood with me through so much pain, I know you share in my relief and happiness today.

Have a great week and God bless.

Your Normal friend,

Donna

The journal readers seemed to breathe that sigh of relief with me.

To: donnahicken@firstcoastnews.com
Subject: 'from Donna's Journal'

Dear Donna

Like so many people, I feel that I have an unfair advantage peeking into your life and watching you go through this latest life challenge.. I just want you to know that I have been praying for you and for your children for so long and am so happy to hear that you are once again "normal." CONGRATULATIONS.

You are so right when you say that God has a plan for you, and, so trusting too. I learned that same lesson nearly four years ago, but, I might say, in a much more different situation. I won't bore you with the details, but, give you a brief run down.... at 36 and after 6 years of no children coming, and many, many years of "female" problems, I was on the table for a hysterectomy. I had cleaned out the baby stuff and mentally prepared myself for the "no more baby" lifestyle that awaited us. We had a huge garage sale and gave away EVERYTHING... the crib I slept in as well my first two children, the coveted "buggy" from the North used for strolling the babies...you name it, we got rid of it... Imagine my surprise then, when the GYN who was to perform my surgery that morning walked into the surgery suite still in his street clothes to tell me that no one had checked my blood work. While I lay in my hospital gown with IV's in my arm, he informed me that instead of having a hysterectomy, I was pregnant! Had I not been hooked up, I probably would have fallen off the table.!!!

It was a year of struggles as we had just relocated to JAX and were really having a harder time adjusting than we expected, etc. but, what an awesome, unexpected blessing. Joseph has just celebrated his 3rd birthday in January and is still, just amazing. To say that God had a plan for our family that we were completely unaware of is a minor understatement. He now also has a 15 month old brother... talk about God being full of surprises and having a grand sense of humor... well, I'm sure you understand this.

While I learned my lesson about God having a plan for me, I feel like I ended up with a pretty good deal. I hope and pray that should I ever be confronted with such life threatening illness in myself or my family, I will continue to have such a strong and unwavering faith. Right now, just raising my kids and struggling with the tiny inconvenience of anemia is enough to keep me humble and on my knees!!

Anyway, take care and God bless you and yours. So many people are praying for you that I know of. Be assured of our continued prayers.
Tricia Gardner

To: donnahicken@firstcoastnews.com
Subject:

Donna, I have followed with much interest your progress through the last few months. You see, I was diagnosed in April with breast cancer. I had surgery in May, followed by chemotherapy and radiation. I cheered you on each day and admired your courage. I knew that if you could be on TV almost every night, then I could struggle through the last few months. I, too, was blessed with many caring friends at work and a supportive family. Through it all, I looked forward to seeing you on the news each night. My hair is finally coming in and it's curly!! Never had curls in my life. And although I am not sure what my natural color is these days, I intend to be adventurous. I can always blame it on the "chemo brain."

I am scheduled for follow up mammograms, etc., for next month and although I am happy to be at this point in treatment, I dread wondering about the results of everything. I was happy to read that your reports were good.
Congratulations!

Today's my birthday (55 years). My friends have showered me with gifts and celebrations all day. It has truly been a blessed day!

In celebration of this day, I wanted to take this opportunity to let you know that you have made a difference in many lives, including mine.
God Bless
Frances Keaton

To: donnahicken@firstcoastnews.com
Subject: 'from Donna's Journal'

That was excellent news today Donna. I'm sure it is more difficult to face the challenges you faced with the whole city watching, but you did an excellent job. I'm sure I speak for all the viewing area. Your good news is good news to everyone, and thanks for being an inspiration (even when you didn't feel like) to everyone.
Mike Daniel

To: donnahicken@firstcoastnews.com
Subject: 'from Donna's Journal'

Hi Donna. I read your journal today and I am sooooo happy for you. I've never been through what you've been through, but I know it must be the toughest thing anyone could possibly want to go through. You've held your head up high and pulled thru it with flying colors. I will continue to pray that you'll never have to battle with this again as long as you live (which will be a long time right????) You are truly an inspiration to all of us!!!!! May the Lord continue to bless you beyond measure...
Your fan,
Carrie Kirkman

To: donnahicken@firstcoastnews.com
Subject: 'from Donna's Journal'

HI Donna,
PRAISE GOD!!! I was so happy to hear your good news. I've never written to you before but I want you to know you have been in my thoughts and prayers. I know first

hand how God can answer prayers. He IS an AWESOME GOD!! I also wanted to let you know I love your hair short. But then you can wear your hair any ole way and look great. I don't get to see the news much on TV but I keep up with the world on line and I so much enjoy your journal. You take care Donna.
Allison Brown (Starke, FL)

To: donnahicken@firstcoastnews.com
Subject: 'from Donna's Journal'

Donna,
Isn't Target a great store? Congratulations on your diagnosis! Just a suggestion, I really like the short hair. I know it's not by design at this point, but it looks great. Have you had your "Wig Burning Party" yet? That should be cathartic. I would wish you good luck, but it sounds like you don't need it anymore. Good luck anyway.
George Ricketson IV

To: donnahicken@firstcoastnews.com
Subject: Thanks !!!

I just wanted to thank you for your willingness to share your "adventure" with a disease that has caused people to cringe at the mere name of it. I have seen it's toll on many members of my family and to know that you are doing so much better fills my heart with great joy.
Thank you again for not only, not running and hiding, but for your openness and your hope.
May God bless you and may you continue to do well.
Virginia Thomas

To: donnahicken@firstcoastnews.com
Subject: Normal

For someone that had a name for her hairpiece, (Brenda. wasn't it?) I think "normal" is a little off the mark. Terrific, Fantastic, SEXY, regular swell person, blessed, and several others are much more accurate than bland ol', 'normal'.
To quote a well-known alien; Live long and prosper.
All love to you and yours,
Libby & Len Wells, down south in St Augustine

To: donnahicken@firstcoastnews.com
Subject: 'from Donna's Journal'

Hi Donna... I am so glad to hear your health is on the upswing. Your bright smile and warm personality is the highlight of my day. Seeing you on the evening news everyday, knowing all that you have been through is one of those thousand points of light former President Bush spoke of a few years ago. I just went through a breast cancer scare with my wife. The first exam was so shocking, they told her they had seen something unusual, and need to do more tests. She had just lost her stepfather and her mother was on her last year of life also, she was confined to her bed and my wife was her caretaker. All this nearly destroyed her. Thank God everything has turned out fine... so far !!!!. She has since lost her mother also and her mind and heart is still very weak. I love her so much and worry everyday about her. She is scheduled for another check up, the dreaded 6 months thing, next week. She is so scared. But she makes it a point to watch you everyday, and is full of smiles when you come on. She was thrilled to see you without your wig, knowing you're getting better each day. I know you must get tons of e-mail like this, so I won't keep you much longer. You are dear in our hearts

and we wish you continued success, and thanks so much for being the strength for so many women in Jacksonville. Donna you are a true ANGEL.
Guy and Sharon Smith

To: donnahicken@firstcoastnews.com
Subject: Donna

Hi, Donna! It is soooo good to hear you doing so well...nobody can deny the strength of prayer, with all that have gone out to you!

I'm still fighting... I am having to put my mom and dad BACK into assisted living this week (the third time) but this is the first time that I have forced them to go - makes me feel sooo guilty but they are just not able to do at home and refuse to have enough help at home, so I had no choice. I think my mother is beginning to get symptomatic now from the lung cancer and wonder if she has some mets to the brain. She is so difficult, irrational - I don't know if it's mets, stubborn, or just plain mad... My dad has failed so that he has forgotten how to perform his regular activities (wash his hair, make a sandwich, etc.)... The whole thing is really sad. My depression is such that I am having a hard time functioning myself, with my health issues (fibromyalgia and probable MS). I guess God will get us all straight somehow. On top of it all Bill and I have both had this cold thing going around (not a big deal but enough already) and then he got bad seafood Sat. and was sick all night and half of Sunday.

The good news is my three baby birds are out of the nest flying around, they have had singing lessons from their mom and dad (not kidding, that was Friday) - they all five sat on a twig-like branch in the cage and mimicked their mom and dad until they got it right. The father has a mop-top hairdo, like a messy skater cut, and one of the baby's has it also!!! When old enough, I am going to get the baby a wife and see if this passes to the NEXT generation. He is so cute (his name is Mop-Top). My Society finches are sitting on four eggs and should hatch about Feb. 8 to 10. We will be away but they are good parents so I'm not worried about them.

Well, again, so nice to hear you are relaxing and getting stronger and doing so well... you and Tim are such a big part of our home - last people we see before we go to bed at night...you're so much like family I don't bother to clean before you come in every night!

Take care and keep up the good feelings - give Tim our best.
Best of all, your hair-do is darling, very sleek and very becoming...you are looking great!
Love,
Patti Thompson

To: PattiThompson
Subject: Your e-mail

Hi Patti!
Goodness girl... you are dealing with a lot. I am so blessed that you still find the energy to give to me. I want you to know that I pray for you often and I'm sending you miles of positives vibes as well. You are such a sweet person...and you have been one of my faithful and constant friends through all of my trials and tribulations. Please don't lose heart through all of this. I can only imagine how difficult it is to see your parents begin to fade mentally. How sad indeed. It's hard to understand God's plan sometimes... but you seem to have a perfect

attitude. Please know that any time you need to vent...
I'm here! Keep singing with the birds sweetie... this too
shall pass.
Love,
Donna

My sweet Patti Thompson. Of all the women, men and children who were my constant companions through this ordeal, Patti was the one with whom I developed the deepest connection. She seemed to know what I was thinking before I did. If I was having a bad day, she could tell instantly. I'd sit down to my computer and there was a note from her.

"OK, what's up? Something's the matter." On good days, she was always the first to notice my smile. I couldn't wait to share things with her. Patti had so much stress in her life. Like me, laughter was her release.

Patti Thompson's Story
by Katrina Mims-Cook

"I'm out of fingers," Patti says jokingly. She splays her fingers on the table for emphasis.

Vibrantly polished fingernails accent several family heirloom ring sets.

"This is my mother's first engagement ring, from 1941, and this is my great grandmother's wedding ring," Patti says displaying several pieces of jewelry hanging from her necklace.

For 59 year-old Patti Thompson, laughter is the best medicine.

"I'm the kind of person, I try to inject humor. I'm like my godmother. She could find something funny no matter what was going on."

Born in Baltimore, Maryland and currently living in St. John's County, just north of St. Augustine, Patti was a medical

233

transcriptionist for St Vincent's Hospital until the sudden illness of her husband Craig forced her into early retirement.

"I nursed him at home the whole time. He didn't want anybody in the house, Hospice or anybody." Craig died 16 weeks after he was diagnosed with lung cancer at the age of 53.

Patti has not remarried, but in 2005, she and her companion, Bill, will have been together long enough to be common-law husband and wife. Bill was diagnosed with prostate cancer five years ago.

"I guess that's why I remember one e-mail in particular Donna sent me. She said she just curled up in a chair and cried. She didn't think she should be doing that. I wrote back and just gave her hell.

I said, "Well you know, why wouldn't you do that with all you're going through? I mean you're bound to break down. That's only human nature."

Shortly after Bill was successfully treated for prostate cancer, Patti took on the responsibility of caring for her mother and her ailing father.

"Amazing Grace, that's what we called her," Patti says, speaking affectionately of her mother, Grace Romoser.

"She was 80 years old when she started chemotherapy and she was having a terrible time with it. She didn't want to talk about it. She wouldn't let me go to the doctor with her. She just didn't want to upset me."

Grace was diagnosed with bladder cancer that had spread to her lungs. This was at about the same time Donna was going through her second bout with breast cancer.

Grace refused to discuss her illness with her daughter, simply saying, "Patti, I don't want to talk about that." Still, she couldn't hide the physical effects of the chemotherapy.

Patti turned to Donna's on-line journal as an outlet.

"You couldn't even discuss cancer with my mother. So I just started writing to Donna. I consoled her in the way I would have consoled my mother."

During all of this, Patti's father's health began a quick decline

234

as well.

"There was just so much going on and I could share this with Donna. We picked each other up. I would tell her about my mother, how frustrated I would get because she wouldn't let me help her. Donna had lost her father so we just bounced off of each other."

Patti's mother Grace passed away on July 1, 2003. Her father, Bill, died two months later on September 15.

Patti is moved to tears when she recalls a gesture of Donna's friendship.

"We had my mother's funeral and when I came home there was a huge basket of flowers by my front door that she had sent. I can't tell you what that did to me when I saw those flowers, with all that she had been through herself."

Patti's been through a lot with her own health recently. Her doctors have been unable to conclusively determine if she has Lupus or Multiple Sclerosis. In spite of her own stress, Patti still has the strength to encourage Donna and make her laugh with funny anecdotes and stories.

"I would e-mail her and say something off-the-wall and she would e-mail me back. I looked forward to her e-mails and she looked forward to mine."

Patti fondly recalls one Christmastime e-mail exchange with Donna.

"I sent her an e-mail when they had the thing on about the man that's building the house and all the profits are going to her Foundation and the BellSouth ladies that got together and did the Christmas presents for the gals she's helping. She always looks so amazed that people are doing this. I wrote to her and I said, "You just don't realize it's just that your sweetness comes through and you're down to earth and you're just a people person and people want to do those things for you." Donna wrote me back and said, "I like you better when I have to give you grief about something.""

Patti says her light-hearted exchanges with Donna are such a gift. As a token of her appreciation, she made Donna a quilt.

"I chose a red brick pattern called Lucky Star. I'm going to put a note on the back where you sign it that says, 'We thank our lucky stars for you in our life.'"

Patti offers the same kindness and encouragement to others in her life. In September of 2003 after checking into several Red Hat Societies in the Jacksonville area, she decided to start her own.

"Some were all breast cancer survivors. Some were all quilters. Some were too big. So I just started my own and I'm the Queen Mother of that group," she says laughing.

Patti's group started with four women, all over the age of 50 with elderly parents and suffering from the empty nest syndrome. As of January 2004, there are 18 members.

"In fact, my first meeting was two days after I buried my father. I'd set the thing up so I thought, well the only thing to do is just go on and go through with it. The girl who was going to help me, her mother died the day before so there was only myself and three other gals there, but there was this instant connection."

The idea for the Red Hat Society comes from a poem a woman in England wrote.

"She said when she was old she was going to wear a red hat and wear purple even though she didn't look good in purple and she was going to eat pickles and do different things," Patti laughs at the thought.

Laughter continues to be her best defense against the stress in her life. Just one more thing that she believes she and Donna have in common.

"I had a lot to share with Donna and she had a lot to share with me. We were going through different things, but we were both coping with so much at once. This bond just formed."

*   *   *

For me, the definition of stress is that which I bury deep inside, try to keep down. There is no physical stress that I find unbearable. Painful maybe, draining, exhausting, but not unbearable. Severe mental stress is another matter entirely. I believe it kills.

236

It's insidious because over time it builds, one block on the next and I don't realize how heavy it's become. It's just something I get used to lugging around. It becomes part of me.

I didn't realize how heavy the weight of those impending tests was, until they were done.

Edith and I have had many conversations about the relationship between stress and cancer. She doesn't believe such a relationship exists. My gut tells me different.

"It's not possible, Donna. The body has a very efficient way of dealing with stress. There are so many chemical reactions that happen as coping mechanisms. It couldn't have caused your cancer."

"But certainly stress compromises the immune system," I argued.

"Cancer is not caused by a failure of the immune system," she countered.

I am clearly no doctor. But, like most women, I have this little voice that tells me when something is amiss with my body. At the time of my first diagnosis, I was under enormous mental stress. Not like the stress of waiting for a test. Sustained, long term, self-imposed stress.

There were things going on in my life that I was trying desperately to control but could not.

I was living in two worlds and they didn't, couldn't connect.

One night, shortly before my diagnosis I had a horrible vicious dream.

I was lying on the floor in a room that was all white. A madman had me bound and gagged. He was using a knife to trace a word on my stomach. The word was an enigma to me. I had never seen it.

T-r-i-c-h-o-t

The next morning, worn out from my dream, I remembered the word distinctly. I looked it up in the dictionary. The closest thing I could find was the word trichotomy: the separation of mind, body and spirit.

I know it sounds crazy and maybe it is. Maybe it's my upbringing, my religion, or just my own paranoid brain.

I have asked myself the question a million times.

"Did I cause my own cancer?"

By pure scientific logic, I suppose the answer is no.

My gut tells me different.

SIXTEEN

Building A Firm Foundation

The Bank of America tower is Jacksonville's tallest building. Visible from both the north and south banks of the St. Johns River, its dark reflective glass drives the eye to its peak 617 feet above the ground.

I glanced at my watch as I made the descent from the Mathews Bridge to downtown.

I've got ten minutes.

My dreams for the Foundation were waiting at the top.

I parked in the massive garage, took one elevator to ground level and a second to the 31st floor.

I spotted the doors to my left. I was told the meeting would take place in the conference room inside.

"Good morning, Donna."

"Hi Steve, wow, what a view!"

Steve Prom looked over his shoulder as if he'd forgotten.

From the long panoramic windows, all of Jacksonville was visible.

"How do you get any work done in here? I'd be staring out the window all day."

Steve smiled. From the looks of things they got plenty of work done. This was no modestly priced attorney's office.

The door opened behind us.

Julie, and her brother Craig Dewhurst entered the room. Craig owns a very successful State Farm insurance office and is involved in tons of charity work. Behind them, my other childhood friend

Celeste Beale, and my cancer survivor buddy Susan Mehrlust filed in.

"Hello everyone, why don't we grab some sandwiches and we'll get down to business," Steve instructed.

Andrea joined us moments later and we all took a seat at a large conference table that ran the length of the room.

Many people had counseled me on the make-up of my board for the Foundation. "You need to get the movers and shakers on board," my Uncle told me. "That's how you raise your money." But I wanted people on this board who had the same passion for the cause that I did. People who I knew and trusted never to misrepresent me, or what the Foundation was about. Besides these friends were no slouches. All were successful business people.

Edith had already agreed to be on the board, but couldn't attend the meeting because of all of her travels. As one of the top breast cancer specialists in the country, she spends much of her time flying all over the globe to lecture on the latest research and clinical trial developments.

Later we would add Bonnie Solloway to the board. Bonnie is a Vice President and Director of Programming for Jacksonville's Gannett stations. She works with me at First Coast News. She and I have always shared a bond. Bonnie has long curly hair which she alternately loves and hates, an eye for fashion and a head for business. She flat out knows how to get things done. I wanted her to help us specifically with corporate fund raising.

"Now that I've called you all here…" I began in a falsely serious voice.

"What are you going to do with us?" Julie completed the thought.

We laughed, but it was a good question.

I knew what I wanted to accomplish. How I was going to do it was still a bit of a mystery.

I turned to Steve.

"How should we proceed?"

"Well, you are going to need a mission statement, but it would

240

be best to start by naming officers."

I looked around the table. No one said a word.

"OK," Steve continued, "Donna you should be the President. You'll also need to name a Secretary and a Treasurer. And you need a CPA."

"I talked with Susie Slappey," Celeste said. "She's in the middle of about a dozen charity projects right now, but she's in. She says just give her a couple of months to get everything else cleared away." Susie is another Bishop Kenny High School buddy. She helps run a very successful family business and she can never say no to a worthy cause.

"Great," Steve said. "It will take at least that long to get everything up and running."

"Celeste, you are a natural to be the treasurer." I said.

She nodded.

Celeste is a Financial Planner for Charles D. Hyman and Company. She's got a big heart and a hard edge. If you want someone to dispense with the small talk and tell it like it is, Celeste is your woman.

When I was first diagnosed with cancer, and just wiped out, Celeste called her former sister-in-law down in Marsh Harbour in the Bahamas and told her we absolutely had to have her home there ASAP for a girl's get away. We were there.

"You'll need to set up a Foundation bank account," Steve said.

Celeste immediately started taking notes.

"I will talk with Marty Lanahan over at AmSouth today about setting up an account."

"Good."

"Julie, why don't you take the Secretary post," I said.

"Wait a minute, I'm no dummy. That means I do all the work right?"

"No, we all do the work. But you are the most organized of anyone at this table."

"OK, Donna, I'll do it under one condition. Show me your purse."

I call my purse the black hole. Things go in, but they rarely come out.

I pulled it up from beside my chair and laid it on the table. As usual, it was overflowing with little scraps of paper, stuffed everywhere. That's how I keep notes. It drives Julie crazy.

"Starting today," she said, "You get all these little pieces of paper out of here and you buy yourself an organizer. Do we have a deal?"

"Deal," I said narrowing my eyes at her. "You drive a hard bargain."

"I'll be the social chairman," Andrea offered. "You know I can plan a party girlfriend."

It's true, but it is far from Andrea's only strength. She once owned a vibrant home contracting business that she built from the ground up. She is also as loyal as it gets with a gift for seeing things from other's perspectives. She is as unselfish as a human being can be and I knew she would personally feel the pain of the women we served.

"And Donna, you know what I want to do most is to talk with the women, give them support," Susan added.

"No one could be better at that," I agreed.

Susan was a high school physical education teacher. She has kind brown eyes and a smile that announces "I love life!" Despite her ongoing cancer battle she seems to have more energy than all of us put together.

Before my eyes, I have personally seen her transform people with her optimism. Her gift for spreading hope is priceless.

She has offered many times to counsel for other cancer survivor groups only to be told she needed to be cancer free for a certain amount of time before she could qualify. I knew for certain their loss would be our gain.

"I'll start getting together all the insurance we need," Craig said. Craig had done this kind of work for other foundations and I knew he'd be right on top of what we had to have. In addition to that he knows everyone in the world. Yes everyone. And he knows how to get what he wants.

For the next two hours, we laid the groundwork for the Foundation.

When Steve got through his list, he looked up.

"Does anyone have any questions or concerns?"

"About a thousand," I said. "But there is one at the top of my list. I don't want this board deciding who qualifies for assistance and who doesn't. I certainly know I don't want to make those decisions. Would it be alright for us to partner with a social service agency like Catholic Charities to screen our potential recipients?"

"Absolutely," Steve said. "Why don't you contact them, and we'll talk about it at the next board meeting in, say, three weeks."

Steve gave us a list of things to do and sent us on our way.

As we made our way out, I asked Julie to stay behind and walk with me to the car.

"Listen Jules," I said. "I know we are an all volunteer army right now, but when this thing is up and running, I mean really running, I want you to consider directing it."

Julie manages a diagnostic center and has a long history in the medical field.

She looked at me as if I was speaking another language.

"Think about it Jules, you're a natural. All those years of dealing with patients and doctors, and now all the contacts you have in the diagnostic community. You could sell ice to the Eskimos, I know you can raise money for a cause you believe in. Most importantly you love me, and I know you want this to be successful as much as I do."

"Oh sure, throw out the emotional blackmail, you know I'm a sucker for that. Actually, it doesn't sound like a bad idea down the road. Let's get started and see how it goes."

"Good, now I've got to go make a phone call," I said.

"Fundraising already?"

"No, I've got to call Cynthia Montello."

"The lady who e-mails you?"

"Yes, I've got a feeling she's going to be an incredible resource in all of this. She owns an ad agency, and she's a cancer survivor, and she's been on top of this project from the moment I first mentioned it."

"Sign her up!"

Without ever having spoken a word to Cynthia Montello, I already knew she was a good soul. She had e-mailed me a half dozen times to see how I was progressing with the Foundation and was anxious to help.

I was ashamed of how long it took me to get my act together, so I was bound and determined not to call until we had actually named the board.

I found the scrap of paper with her number on it and dialed.

"The Montello Agency."

The woman on the other end of the phone sounded British.

"May I speak with Cynthia Montello please?"

"May I ask who's calling?"

"It's Donna Hicken."

"One moment please."

The woman put me on hold, and in seconds Cynthia picked up.

"So, we finally speak," she said in a low mellow voice that would put most radio disc jockeys to shame.

"Finally," I said. "I just wanted you to know that we put our board together today and I really want you to be part of this Foundation. I can't tell you how much your support has egged me on to get this done."

"God puts people together for a reason," she replied. "What can I do?"

"Can you design a logo?"

"I certainly can. What is the name of the foundation?"

"The Donna Hicken Foundation," I said, with a cut line underneath. "Caring for women living with breast cancer."

"I'll get right on it."

Cynthia and I met a couple of weeks later to go over the logo designs and get to know each other better.

She would have been totally justified in being irritated with me. I had doubled her workload, scrapping her first logo design at the last minute, and then drawing a crude sketch of the symbol I had in mind. She had to start all over and she was doing all of this for free.

I settled on an image of two women, holding their arms up in triumph with a heart and pink breast cancer ribbon between them.

"It's no trouble at all," she said sincerely. "This is small next to the things we're going to do with this Foundation."

"I hope you're right," I said.

Cynthia Montello's Story
by Tonn Pastore

"I treated cancer from the start until the finish as if it were nothing more than something on my appointment book. I never gave it thought. I never gave it time. I never gave into it. I never felt sorry for myself. I don't remember ever crying about it at all. I literally treated it like it was a meeting or something I had to show up for."

Cynthia Montello leans forward behind her desk. Her clear hazel eyes and full smile are enough to get one's attention, but it's her voice, clear and melodic that makes folks stop and listen.

In 1989 she went to the doctor to have a small lump on her neck investigated. It was dismissed as benign and left alone. A year later Cynthia sprained her back in an aerobics class and returned to the doctor. An x-ray showed a mass that was alarming. Further examination, more x-rays and then a biopsy by a throat specialist, Dr. Lawrence Lisska, revealed she had developed thyroid cancer (papillary carcinoma) and that it spread from her thyroid to her neck and from there to her throat and into her shoulder and chest.

"I remember being alone in the car after I got the news. I felt as if the floor had been pulled out from under me and I came crashing down on my back. All I could think about was my husband and my kids. Nothing mattered but that. I was flooded with so many emotions all at one time that it's really hard to sort it all out. I think I sat in the car for two hours finally pounding on the steering wheel enraged."

She told her husband Howard what the doctor said. With her two little boys, David and Jeff, just six and three at the time, she decided that nothing was going to beat her.

"I guess I got angry. I was so angry, because I was not going to die. The thought of not watching them grow up, the thought of not being able to spend the rest of my life with my husband was, let me put it this way, I refused to accept it. That's exactly how I approached the whole thing. I spent the whole time I had it and getting rid of it with that attitude. My doctor told me later that he thought it was probably that very attitude that caused my body to fight so hard."

The doctors told her there was a chance she would never speak again and likely have to use an artificial voice box. They also prepared her to be unable to use her left arm after the operation on her shoulder.

In spite of this news she made plans for a full recovery. Before the operation, she let go a staff of six people from her thriving advertising agency and moved her office into her home, keeping only a few clients she felt she could handle. She gave up 2 million dollars of business because she knew she couldn't handle it on her own.

In April 1990, Cynthia underwent an eight-hour surgery to remove the cancer. "When I woke up in the recovery room, I said, 'How did I do?' I can remember hearing all these people saying, 'She can't be talking! She can't possibly be talking!'"

Her mother, Suzie and her sister Geri, visited and helped during her recovery but they had to go back to their families. "So mostly it was Howard that took care of our children, the house and me during that time. He was incredible. He'd say 'I never knew you did so much!' He got a quick lesson in balancing a career, children and a home. Every man should go through it. They will gain an appreciation for their wife!"

Howard and Cynthia met while he was vacationing in Myrtle Beach. Cynthia was living there at the same time. Howard was taking a walk on the beach and stopped to ask her the time. Her classic beauty and red hair captivated him. That was 23 years ago. They've been together ever since.

During her recovery in the hospital she received stacks of cards and letters. Howard would come up and read them every night. "All that love from others and all that time Howard spent with me equated into something tangible for me. I never realized love was a tangible resource. That's when it all became real to me. It took cancer to wake me up!"

God had always been an important part of Cynthia's life but now it was different. "My impression of God changed tremendously. It's as if I was awakened spiritually, physically, I mean everything in me changed from that moment. Everything that was important to me was no longer so. I thought God was just a vision of some big guy with white hair and robes and light coming from him. I was always a good Episcopalian. I went to church and all that, but I didn't even know Jesus until all this happened. I was born again in some fashion but I have to tell you how."

Cynthia's focus changes and she lowers her voice. "At some point in the hospital recovery room, my throat cramped and I quit breathing. There was someone in the room and she went to get help. I can only remember asking God to see the face of Jesus. I think I thought I was going to die and I wanted to see His face so that I would feel peace."

Instead of seeing the face of Jesus, what she saw was a lamb. "He put his face right up on the bed and he nudged my hand with his nose. I felt it, I saw it and it was real. It was not fuzzy or blurry not a vision. It was real. Jesus sent the lamb so that I would see him for who he really is. He's the lamb of God."

She found herself trying to tell her friends about this experience. They all seemed to say the same thing. "Well, you were on heavy pain medication, you were dreaming." Or, "Well, it's a metaphor for Christ, your mind just told you that's what you were seeing." So Cynthia stopped telling people that part of her story, until now.

"People ask me, 'Why do you think God healed you and not others?' I don't know why, I just know that He did heal me. It made me understand that God is in every single thing that exists. He exists wholly in every cell, the tip of your eyelash, in every particle, in everything that surrounds us, everything we are. That is where God is, that is where we find God, in those details. He's not some guy that's removed from us. Every act of love makes a difference, every act of evil makes a difference. It's all cumulative."

This change led her to accept an invitation from Raiford State Penitentiary, to go and minister to the AIDS infected prisoners. A work, close to her heart, as her brother Kelly died of AIDS. Cynthia and Davette Turk, an Episcopal priest volunteered to go.

They went and led the evening prayers and services. She sang, they preached and prayed with the men. "I just went and visited with the guys that had AIDS, talked to them and helped them prepare for death. I tried to help them know God, to help them have comfort in their life. My hope was for them to accept the choices they had made, to accept their future however short it was."

She started out with five men and by the time she quit going they had standing room only. "Some say they came to see a woman, but I know, looking out on them with their arms raised to the ceiling, tears pouring down their faces, God was touching them, it wasn't me, it was God."

Cynthia's experiences from singing on the road in rock bands afforded her a true connection to some of the men. "They knew I was real, that I wasn't talking down to them. I'd done some of the same things that had landed them behind bars. The first thing I told them was there was no difference between us, except that I didn't get caught. I made all the mistakes and I'm glad. I look at politicians today and they ask us to vote for them because they're perfect. What kind of leader can someone be, who hasn't made mistakes?"

248

The visits stopped when the priest could no longer go but Cynthia kept up her ministry with the men through correspondence.

Cynthia found strength from her family and did not seek help from groups with similar experience. "All I could think about was when I was 8 months pregnant, every stranger I met told me about the birth of their child. I could get on an elevator and perfect strangers would rub my stomach or tell me about how everything went wrong and they had to have an emergency C-section and it scared me. By the time I had the baby I'd heard every horror story that's out there. I didn't want that to happen again so that made me not talk to anybody who had cancer or seek any kind of support. I knew as long as I didn't give in to it, I knew I was going to be fine."

Her determination was strong enough to have her singing after a year and a half. During this time, she did all the right things including eating a diet that promoted cancer fighting cells and staying away from the "wrong foods."

"I didn't eat a french fry for a year!"

Still a check up in 1994 revealed the cancer had returned. "It's devastating to hear that it isn't gone. You fight so hard to be free of it."

This time doctors gave her a treatment unique to thyroid cancers. Instead of surgery she was placed in an isolated hospital room where she was quarantined for six days. A man in a "space suit" came into the room with a lead container on a metal tray. With tongs he pulled out a box that contained six pills of radioactive iodine.

"After I leave the room, and please wait until I am out of the room, you must open this vial and swallow all six of the pills," he said.

"You want me to swallow something you won't even stand in the same room with?"

"This is your radiation therapy, if you want to get rid of your cancer, you need to take these iodine pills."

Cynthia did as the lead suited man told her and began the six day wait with no physical contact from anyone. She spent her time reading and painting portraits of angels. Two examples hang on the walls of her office today.

The second treatment was successful and a year later in November of 1995 she was declared cancer free. "Today I get a mammogram every year, I watch for sore throats, I check on fatigue and other than Synthroid I don't take any medications.

Now nine years later, during two 90 minute services every Sunday, her voice leads the All Souls Church contemporary band through a half a dozen songs.

From the time she was a little girl learning about music and how to play the harp from her grandmother, Cynthia Montello wanted to be a professional singer. She dreamed of becoming a recording artist and was the lead vocalist in bands that played all over the country.

When her career in rock bands did not pay all the bills, she took a job at an advertising agency in Cincinnati, Ohio. Starting as a receptionist she learned the business from the bottom up. Later moving to Jacksonville, she opened her own advertising business. Today the Montello Agency specializes in advertising for building contractors. "We do all types of advertising, including designing model centers for new construction sites."

Taking care of her health, her family and a growing business have occupied Cynthia's time and energy since her last surgery. Then one day an advertising representative from Channel 12 was in her office and mentioned in passing that Donna Hicken was going to start a foundation for breast cancer.

"It just hit me like a bolt. I knew I had to help her. I didn't even know why. It was just God's prodding I think. I didn't even know her but I told the rep to get me her e-mail address. I wanted to let her know I was available if she needed me. I sent her an e-mail telling her I was a cancer survivor and I owned an ad agency at her disposal. She e-mailed me right back with, 'Are you serious? Are you for real?'

"I think it took several e-mails for her to believe me. I don't

250

think she really thought there was somebody out there like me. It was God again playing all the pieces, moving people and things to be able to bless these women who don't have insurance or money."

Cynthia's rich voice strengthens, "It's unthinkable that somebody has to fight that fight, not having all the resources I had, friends, money, insurance and everything else. There was nothing stopping me from getting the very best care. But if I didn't have that and I had no kids or husband, what would have happened to me? I would have died and nobody would have cared. I knew I had to help."

Like all the other things in Cynthia's life she knows God has a plan. "I've prayed so many times and God has led me down so many roads since then. Donna and I hit it off. She's an incredible, wonderful person. I was happy to do advertising work for the Foundation but that is nothing compared to the need that is out there. We're just scratching the surface right now."

*   *   *

"You will find," Cynthia assured me with her golden voice, "that when you are doing something for good, something that God wants you to do, doors will fly open."

I tried to remember those words as I turned my attention to Catholic Charities.

It is the largest social service organization in the area. The people there are pros and they are compassionate. They are also mind-bogglingly busy and I wasn't sure they'd agree to add another straw to the camel's back. Still, I was convinced they were the key to our success in helping women, and to our credibility in fundraising.

I called the director Bill Beitz and we agreed to meet at a new downtown restaurant and pub called The London Bridge. It was just down the street from both my office and Catholic Charities.

I was nervously rehearsing the words I'd use to make my case, when I spotted Bill at a booth. He smiled and waved me over.

We exchanged our hellos and I launched into my plea.

"So, whatever you could do Bill would be wonderful. I know how busy…."

"We'd be happy to help."

The words left his mouth before I'd even finished.

Bill went on to say that the charity would play as large a role as we found necessary, and that I needn't worry about anything.

I felt tears come to my eyes.

"I thought you might say 'no,'" I said. "And I had absolutely no idea what I was going to do if you did."

"I talked with our board as soon as I got your call. Everyone is in complete support."

"Thank you so much," I said, rising from my seat to give him a much deserved hug."

"I can tell this is very important to you," he said smiling. "Fundraising is a lot of work, but once you have a taste of this, you'll never be able to give it up. How are things going so far?"

"So far, I said, doors are flying open."

SEVENTEEN

Anchors Away

It was May, the middle of ratings. It's a stressful time in the news business. Stations have to perform well because the numbers are used to sell advertising. Everyone is on edge. It's a rule, really. You're not allowed to feel relaxed during a ratings period. If you're not miserable, you must not be working hard enough and if you're not working hard enough, the numbers won't be good.

I'm not used to seeing Mike smile much during ratings. (Rules are rules)

But when I walked into his office, there it was.

"Is that a smile?"

"Have you heard the news?"

That explained it. This was an "I know something you don't know" smile. Those are always permitted.

"Mike, you know I'm always the last one to know anything. What news?"

"Deborah Gianoulis is leaving the anchor desk."

"That is not funny."

"I'm not kidding. She's going to leave news and start producing her own documentaries."

Standing in Mike's office I felt like someone had just put a fist in my gut.

I lowered myself into a chair and stared at him.

"How could she do this to me," I said.

Mike shook his head.

"Come on, Donna, she's been anchoring for almost 25 years. Maybe she's just ready for a change."

253

"But I'M not ready," I said. "No one consulted ME."

Deborah Gianoulis anchored the evening news for the competition. She is my hero. She came to speak to my class when I was a senior in high school and I was instantly impressed. She was the reason I went into broadcasting instead of print journalism. My goal in life was to come home to work in Jacksonville one day and be just like her.

No one could be Deborah of course. She is the most genuine self-effacing person who's ever graced a news desk. As her co-anchor of many years Tom Wills would later say, "To Deborah it was never about celebrity, it was about service."

Much to my delight, we developed a friendship over the years. I found a security in looking up every night to see her on the TV monitors, knowing she was there, working just across the river from me.

I went to my desk and burst into tears. I was actually feeling grief. I knew it was silly. It's not like she had died or anything, but it was the end of an era, one that had defined my youth and my career.

I spent most of the late afternoon watching Channel 4 to see what Deb would say to her viewers. There were several times during my own broadcast that I looked back at the monitors behind me to watch her. At the end of her six o'clock news Deborah announced her decision with her usual class and grace. I was hoping she'd change her mind.

In fact, I gave her a whole day to do it before, resigned, I finally sat down to send her an e-mail.

To: 'DGIANOUL@wjxt.com'
Subject: OUCH!

Well Miss Deborah,
I knew you were going to go and break my heart one day. I missed my tease during the six o'clock show last

night because I couldn't tear my unblinking eyes away from your announcement. All day long I've had this big fat rock in my throat. I know you must be so excited about your new path... and I'm excited for you. But the truth is... I never wanted to look up and not see your smiling face shining from my monitor. As usual, you are the class of the city. I envy your new schedule and look forward to catching more of your documentary work. Say 'hello' to Tom. Probably one person even sadder than me today.

All the best,

Donna

A few minutes later the assignment desk was paging me.

"Donna, Deborah G. is on the phone for you."

I ran to pick up the call.

"OK," she said in a mockingly stern voice. "I made it through the entire day without crying until now. Thanks a lot!"

We both started bawling.

Deborah and I had been planning a walk on the beach from the time of my rediagnosis. Her resignation gave us the push to follow through.

We set a time. She would come to the condo and we'd go from there.

It was a windy gray day, perfect for an undisturbed walk. Aside from the occasional seagull we were alone on the beach.

We hugged and cried and talked about the past and about purpose in life.

"You've always been so optimistic Deb, so positive."

"I've been blessed that way," she said. "It really is how I see the world."

"With documentaries I can help people in a way that I couldn't in television news. Not that what we do on the news desk doesn't help people. It was just time for a new challenge."

"Aren't you scared?"

255

"Of course, that's part of it. But I can do this."

"I wish I had your confidence."

I had earlier confided in Deborah that the thought of tackling a foundation for breast cancer survivors seemed out of my league. She had offered encouragement and advice on people who could help me. On this day, I was feeling particularly vulnerable.

"I want so much for this Foundation to be a success, and I'm so afraid I'm going to fall flat on my face with it," I said.

"You won't Donna. As long as you remember who you are doing it for, you won't fail."

"And one other thing," she said.

"Be grateful."

Grateful.

I turned the word over in my head.

I am grateful. Truly grateful, maybe for the first time in my life.

The word has since become my signature, literally. It's how I sign almost every letter asking for donations or thanking people for them.

Donna's Journal
Home > Health
June 19, 2003

It's been a long time since I've written one of these entries. I hope you'll forgive me. I've been enjoying good health....and also working very hard on a project that I hope you will find very exciting. You have all shown me so much compassion.

I have often told you that your prayers and support truly pulled me through my breast cancer treatment. I believe that support still lifts me every day. I told you all along that I believe God has a plan for me, and while I know that plan is vast, I have gotten a message loud and clear that there is something I must do to pass that compassion along.

Every day on the First Coast two woman are told the news that shatters their lives. They have breast cancer. I know as a mother, my first thought beyond total fear was... dear God, please let me be here to see my babies grow up.

Fortunately for me, I have a well paying job, understanding bosses, good insurance, and a support system second to none.

Many thousands of women don't have that.

In fact, they don't have time to worry about whether they will be here to watch their children grow up... because they are worrying so much about whether they have enough money to keep a roof over their heads.

Cancer itself is so stressful, financial stress on top of that is just that last straw that pushes many women into despair. Whatever time any of us has, it should be spent caring for each other.

So, toward that end, with the help of many people, I am launching The Donna Hicken Foundation. The foundation will raise money to be used exclusively for First Coast women living with breast cancer... who, for whatever reason, can't make ends meet.

For any of you who have ever had a serious illness, you know that even good insurance doesn't cover everything. Costs associated with long term care are immense. Not to mention the fact that mortgages and car payments are still there even if the money is not.

I mentioned this plan to you many months ago... but it is just now coming together. The need is great, but so is the heart of this community. You have shown me that. I ask for your prayers now more than ever, that we can make this a lifeline for many women who need us.

Take care and God bless,
Donna

The news got a warm welcome from the journal readers. I would have expected nothing less. In so many ways, these were the people who taught me to be grateful. Gratefulness, I've learned, is contagious.

To: donnahicken@firstcoastnews.com
Subject: 'from Donna's Journal'

Donna,
I'm glad to see you are doing so much better. I have been following your journal & saying prayers for you. I even e-mailed you once & you answered me ! That was so nice. I commented on how you manage to stay so "chipper" throughout your treatment & how I miss you when you aren't on the air.
I have a friend that has cancer & lost her job. She can't afford Cobra and she's not going to be able to afford her treatments. How would I get more information for her? She is a very proud & stubborn woman. I have to research this because I know she won't do it herself.
Once again, it is so nice to see you on the road to recovery & dedicating your time & effort toward helping others.
Debra Hoffkins

To: donnahicken@firstcoastnews.com
Subject: 'from Donna's Journal'

You Go Girl. I am so proud of you.
Bright Blessings to You,
Nan Gorden (Brunswick, GA)

To:donnahicken@firstcoastnews.com
Subject: 'from Donna's Journal'

Hi Donna,
I am so glad you are doing so good these days. And congrats on a great kick off for the Donna Hicken Foundation. I work in the field of sonography, most recently in The Breast Center, and I have seen lots of cancers, come and go. I believe as you do, God truly has a special plan for you. You have helped so many women get thru the same ordeal. You don't know me, but I feel as if I have known you for 25 years.
You see I knew your grandfather, Rufus, and I have always wanted to tell you something I'm sure you have always known.. He loved you so much....... he talked about you quite often, and man, did he love your children........ I have never wrote anyone like this before, but I had a strong feeling to look up your diary. I've never done that before. I think Rufus wants to say "Hi." I hope somehow this brings a smile to you today Donna, it did me.......
Love to you and yours,
Lori Thomas (St. George, GA)

To: donnahicken@firstcoastnews.com
Subject: Donna Hicken Foundation

Donna,
Congratulations on the start of your foundation! I hope it is an overwhelming success.

As you may know, RE/MAX is a proud sponsor of the Susan G. Komen Breast Cancer Foundation. To that end, I would be willing to donate a portion from every real estate transaction closed to your foundation to assist in breast cancer awareness and research.

Please advise who I should contact to setup this donation effort.
P.S... Tim's brother brokered a few mortgage loans for some of my past clients.
Regards,
Phyllis Staines

To: donnahicken@firstcoastnews.com
Subject: 'from Donna's Journal'

You never cease to amaze me; your light and courage continue to shine through. My prayers are always with you and will continue... please let me know what we, as your angel crew out here, can do to help and get involved! You sure GO GIRL and all of us benefit from your spunk!

My Mom is about the same, maybe not quite as alert, but still has the fight - not fighting the cancer now, but fighting to keep and get everything in order (me, the staff, etc). She has planned her entire funeral (thank heavens that's through - was kind of morbid), had us bring pictures of caskets and picked hers and my Dad's... this is so hard, but try to keep the humor in the situation... The other day she was making her list and checking it twice and called me to find how if her caregivers would remember to feed her if she went in a coma...

On that note I will again say congratulations on your so worthwhile and needed foundation and let me know how I can help... best love to you and your family...
Patti Thompson

To: Patti
Subject: 'from Donna's Journal'

Hi Patti,
You sweetheart... it breaks my heart to read your note. I'm so so sorry about your mom. I remember so well having to make similar decisions about my dad and I still can't think about it without crying. Thank you for your unrelenting support as always. If you will send me your address I will send you an invitation to our kickoff fundraiser next week. It's a dinner at a new restaurant in Neptune Beach called Sunny Caribee. Should be fun. It's next Thursday the 26th. And believe me... I will take all the help I can get with all of this stuff. I'm so afraid someone is going to walk in one day and say... "what? you let HER do that? I feel totally overwhelmed... but the support has been amazing. Further confirmation for me that this is the path God wants me to walk. Hang in there walking yours too sweetie. If I can do anything beyond pray... please let me know. I will definitely be praying. God bless...and don't forget to send me your address! Please give your mom my love.
Donna

I was hoping others would be as gracious.

A version of that journal entry went out on invitations announcing the Foundation's first fundraiser. A dinner at the Sunny Caribee Restaurant in Neptune Beach.

Once again, as Cynthia predicted, doors were flying open.

We didn't pay for anything. The restaurant donated all the food. The wine and beer were donated. Cynthia even managed to get the printing for free.

Marsha Burroughs was the manager at Sunny Caribee. A petite

blonde islander, Marsha has an easy confidence about her.

She seemed amused by my need to worry.

"What if we run out of food?"

"We won't," she said smiling.

"What if people don't come?"

"They will."

Finally, one night, after I rang her home phone for about the eighth time that evening she set me straight.

"Donna," she said, her voice full of assurance, "don't you know that God's hands are all over this? Stop worrying."

I had to smile.

Marsha's words reminded me so much of Cynthia's.

They also reminded me of my preacher friend Tawana Tuggles.

Tawana is a high-spirited African American woman who became my friend years ago after she won a community service award from the station. She fights enormous physical challenges, but she claims never to worry.

"I don't worry," she says, "I pray. If you're going to worry, don't pray. If you're going to pray, don't worry."

Easier said than done.

I had no trouble praying, but I still worried.

Marsha met me at the door to the restaurant.

"Let's have fun," she said. "It's going to be great."

She pressed something into my hand.

"You need this more than I do tonight," she said.

I looked down and saw a small silver guardian angel medallion. It didn't leave my hand the entire evening.

First Coast News photographer Steve Berrios motioned to me from across the street.

"Ready for you Donna. We've got about five minutes. The producer wants to see you in front of the camera."

Mike agreed to let me anchor the early evening shows from Sunny Caribee.

"Donna Hicken is live in Neptune Beach tonight to tell us about the start of something big to help women with breast cancer on

262

the First Coast."

"Thanks Alan, I'm here in Neptune Beach to celebrate the start of The Donna Hicken Foundation. The Foundation has my name for fundraising purposes, but this Foundation belongs to the women in our area living with breast cancer, who are struggling to make ends meet."

The response was overwhelming. Before the party even started, people were driving by, handing me money in the street. One man gave me three hundred dollars.

The event itself was a beautiful blur. The restaurant was packed. People were incredibly generous. Even the waiters and waitresses donated their tips.

So many good friends, who didn't have the time, took it anyway.

Former F.S.U. and Green Bay Packer star Leroy Butler came by to donate a portion of his book sales.

Tom Coughlin, the former Jaguars coach, and his wife Judy were there too. Their daughter Keli was the first person I turned to when I was trying to set up the Foundation because of her huge success running the Jay Fund, Tom's charity for leukemia patients. It was Keli who first made me believe this night was even possible.

Gary Mack, a well-known local artist donated a framed print to be auctioned off.

Edith was there, and Dr. Reimer, who first tried to make sense of my brain.

All of my family and Tim's, my kids. It was intoxicating.

Most amazing though was the scores of people who showed up that I didn't know. People who just believed in what we were doing and wanted to help.

Marsha stood beaming in the corner.

"I told you," she said.

The event was meant as an introduction as much as a fundraiser. We went in thinking we'd be extremely fortunate to raise four or five thousand dollars.

When the night was over and the last dollar counted, we had raised more than ten thousand.

Celeste and Julie brought me a glass of wine.

"Let's have a toast," Celeste said.

"To the beginning of a legacy that will be here serving others long after we're gone."

We clinked glasses.

"YA YA," Celeste shouted, laughing in reference to the famous sisterhood of childhood friends.

"YA YA," Julie and I repeated.

To: donnahicken@firstcoastnews.com
Subject: Thursday's Foundation Kickoff

Dear Donna,

I just wanted to say how much I admire you and your desire and passion to make the world a better place. My husband, neighbor, and I zoomed down to the beach after hearing just the tail-end of Thursday afternoon's newscast and your spot on the benefit. We didn't even get exactly where it was - just the Neptune Beach part. So, we went into the bookstore across the street and a kind customer shopping directed us to the right spot.

The glass of wine was lovely, but the wonderful part was seeing so many people supporting such an important cause. I felt like a groupie or something, and am pretty shy by nature, but I felt I just had to speak to you, so I waited until Coach Coughlin and his wife finished greeting you, then I mumbled something to you. You were so very gracious, just as I would have imagined, and asked for my name and number to know who was in attendance. We were going for a walk on the beach and intended to return before 9 p.m., but we didn't get back in time.
Becky Anding

To: donnahicken@firstcoastnews.com
Subject: P.S.

Donna, four of the teachers at my school have had Breast Cancer in the past five years and several of my friends. I know how devastating it can be, and thank you from the bottom of my heart for being so open, honest, and inspirational with your cancer, both times. You are truly a very special lady, and I will continue to support the foundation in any way that I can. Best wishes and God bless.
Sincerely,
Becky Anding

Weeks later, the money continued to roll in, and the Foundation served its first recipient.

Lisa, a young mom, was dealing with a recurrence of her breast cancer. She was beside herself with worry over her children and her finances.

The Foundation paid her bills. In her words "a huge burden lifted" from her shoulders.

Julie talked with her on the phone, and then called me crying.

"Get used to it," I said. "You're going to be crying a lot. But that's not such a bad thing."

"Oh no, I'm not upset," she said still sniffing. "It's just that she was so..... so Grateful."

Grateful.

EIGHTEEN

Run For Your Life

On October 12, 2003, a year and a lifetime later than we planned, Tim and I ran the Chicago Marathon.

I ran as slow as mud. Slower. But it was one of the most satisfying races I've ever run.

Of course the week before we left for Chicago I came down with the worst cold I'd had in a year. It developed into bronchitis after several days and I placed a frantic call to Edith who was in New York for a presentation.

"I'm coughing up green stuff and I only have four days before the race," I said.

"I suppose you want to run."

"I'm GOING to run."

"OK, let's get you on some antibiotics."

The whole scene reminded me of a funny conversation I had years ago with Bill Rodgers. If you are a runner, Bill needs no introduction. He is a four time Boston Marathon winner. He comes to Jacksonville every year to run in the Gate River Run 15k National Championship, and won it the first year it was in existence. Bill has electric blue eyes and wild strawberry blonde hair that sticks straight up and he has the most incredible love for running. He's a blast to be around.

"Everyone comes down with something before a race," Bill said. "It's our built-in excuse to run poorly. My leg hurts, or my foot hurts...."

"So what's wrong with you?" I asked.

"My knee hurts," he said, his mischievous eyes sparkling.

It's so true, although I suspect there is probably some science involved. No one just steps out and runs 26 miles. Even slowly. It takes long hours of running. Many athletes will get in 60 or 70 miles in a week, just to prepare. So invariably, your body starts talking to you. Fatigue and sometimes injury, or as in my case, a bad cold. The smart runners learn to cross train. A little less running, a little more swimming or biking. I've never had the discipline to do it. I will swim or bike if forced by injury, but to me, there is nothing in the world like taking off on my own two legs, just me and the road and the world. There is nothing else that gives me the same freedom and focus.

I knew it was going to be an emotional day before the race ever started.

Scores of runners were lined up at the port-a-potties for that one last nervous pee before the start. I struck up a conversation with a nice woman named Emily who had run ten marathons in ten years. This would be her 11th.

"Pretty impressive to stay injury free long enough to do that many in a row," I said.

"I'm celebrating my 11th year of life after breast cancer," she said.

I walked into the john and swallowed hard, wanting to push the tears down along with the lump in my throat.

"Save it for the race, Donna," I thought.

But I had so much inside, I could have run a hundred marathons and still had plenty of emotion to spare.

Tim and I exchanged a last hug well before the start.

"Have a beautiful run," he said. "I'll be waiting at the finish."

"You'd better be," I teased. "And try to at least look like you're still a little sweaty. I know you'll have time for a shower and dinner by the time I get in, but restrain yourself."

"Stop it. You know the goal. Just finish."

He went to join the corral of "preferred" starters.

I placed myself in front of a big round yellow sign that read "5 hour pace."

I have never been one to set land speed records, but I always run hard. Still, Tim was right. This time I just wanted to celebrate my way to the finish.

It was fun to listen to the conversations around me. Many first time marathoners anticipating the race. Wondering if they could really make it.

And one man, who had run the Chicago Marathon 25 times!

"I think I've finally got a pretty good grasp of the course," he said.

The course is a picturesque history of downtown Chicago.

The starting line is on Columbus Drive. It's in the middle of Grant Park, right on Lake Michigan. The area is known as "Chicago's front yard." The knick-name sounds welcoming, and it fits. Sailboats dot the lakefront as people stroll and jog along a well-manicured path. It could be a scene in Florida, only instead of pelicans, it's geese that fly in formation overhead.

When the gun sounded it took my group 21 minutes to get to the start line. As we inched our way forward in a mash of runners, I was chatting with a woman named Lorraine from Fort Lauderdale.

"I've run nine marathons and every time I finish my husband buys me a piece of jewelry," she said. "This year I finish, I get diamonds."

"I guess you'll finish."

"Never failed yet."

Lorraine and I spent the first mile weaving in and out of runners, barely able to move. Then we each went our own way.

I ran the rest of the race alone, with 40,000 of my closest friends.

Maybe it's because I was taking time to enjoy the sights, but I have never seen such incredible crowd support in any race. I'm told a million people lined the course.

Spectators were five or six deep, practically the entire 26.2 miles.

One of my favorite spots was between miles 9 and 10, an area called Lincoln Park.

Like much of the area, it had been destroyed by the great Chicago fire of 1871, but quickly rebuilt. Beautiful homes line the streets, with trees which are absolutely bursting with golden leaves. The last celebration of color before Chicago's bitter winter takes hold. People were so close along the sides, it felt as if they were sweeping me along.

I high-fived every kid with a hand out, and twisted wildly as a band played "The Twist" at mile 13. As we passed Greektown just after the halfway mark, I nearly had my eye poked out by a woman with a flag, who bent down to pick up her camera. I also found myself running beside some of the craziest folks I've ever seen. Of course many people would argue that anyone willing to run this far without being chased is crazy, but this was a great mix of humanity.

There were three guys who looked to be in their 20s, running side by side in matching T-shirts. The back of one shirt said, "he's not heavy," the next shirt continued, "he's my brother." The third added, "my brother too."

A group of women I'd place in their 50s wore bumble bee costumes with bobbing antennae on the their heads. Some younger ladies were dolled up with glittery T-shirts that read "team fabulous." The crowd loved them.

The rowdiest folks by far were in the Pilsen's Hispanic area. Spectators hung from balconies, and lined the streets waving Mexican flags and screaming encouragement at the top of their lungs. Colorful murals depicting Hispanic culture were everywhere. Any runner carrying a Mexican flag was lauded with thunderous applause.

It was perfect timing. Mile 20, people were starting to drag, and the temperature was approaching 70°, warm by marathon standards.

I ran by one man who I would have sworn was walking unconscious in a full Winnie the Pooh costume. All that was visible was his round sweaty face with dark swirls of hair dripping down from below Winnie's head.

Tim would later have the best tale though. A guy he ran by during the race was simply wearing his underwear. Not boxers, jockeys. In magic marker he had scribbled on his back this announcement: "the 11th commandment - don't make bets with friends while drunk."

My trainer and friend Brett Chepenik had asked me to write two things on my sneakers.

"YCDI" and "YUC."

The letters stood for "You Can Do It" and "Yes U Can."

"If I slow down enough to read that, I'll be in trouble," I told him.

As it turned out I didn't need to. People all along the way held out signs and shouted those very words of encouragement.

My mind flashed back to the Boston Marathon in 1999 and all the little bald cancer patients from The Dana-Farber Cancer Institute out waving us on. "Go Dana-Farber," they screamed as we ran by in our charity singlets. It made me cry then and of course it made me think about my own healthy children. Nothing could be more devastating than having a child go through that hell. I couldn't imagine doing that race now that I had experienced cancer.

"Go Donna Hicken!"

The cheers from a spectator from Jacksonville forced my thoughts back to the present. I waved and gave a big thumbs up.

I am not going to lose it today.

I don't know why that thought was so stuck in my head. For the better part of a year now I had been storing it all up. The frustration. The fear. The pain. The anger. The hope.

It was all right there just beneath the surface. I'd been fighting tears for days.

Let it all go.

But I couldn't. I was soaking in the scene, but I think I feared if I let the floodgates open I'd never stop. I was using all of that emotion as fuel.

As I rounded mile 21 a band was playing the tune "No Time Left For You." I was on a pace to finish about 4:45 but I had to laugh. Somehow, time evaporates between miles 20 and 26. I don't know how, it just does.

When I ran the Disney Marathon in 1998, I thought at mile 18, I had a great shot at 3:45. That would qualify me for Boston, the

271

only marathon for which runners must qualify unless they are racing for a charity (like Dana-Farber). But after mile 20, each mile took me a little longer. I couldn't figure it out. I had pushed through the worst part physically at about mile 17 and felt good, but there it was. In the end, my time was 3:56:40. Respectable for an average runner like me, but not good enough to qualify.

It's interesting how cancer redefines success.

"Are you going to win Mommy?" Drew always asks me this question before I race.

Usually I just toss back something like "not this time Drew, but I'll keep trying."

Now I answered differently.

"That depends on your definition of winning, Drew. If I finish, I win."

After surviving two bouts with breast cancer, just to finish at all in Chicago sounded like victory to me.

I can't tell you much about the last five miles of the race. I was heavy duty into my rosary by then, counting on each mystery to get me to the next mile.

Tim would later talk about how much he enjoyed running by Comiskey Park at mile 23. I don't remember seeing it at all.

My mouth had gone completely dry from all the anti-histamines and my muscles felt shredded. Despite my best efforts to hydrate before the race, the medications had dried me out pretty badly.

After some final twists and an evil little hill, added in the last half mile, I was finally on Michigan Avenue. I could see the balloons and banners that marked the finish. People in the grandstands were cheering loudly. I put what was left of my legs in gear and pushed it home.

The race ended almost exactly where it began in Grant Park.

I crossed the finish line in 5:01:48, more than a full hour and five minutes slower than that day in Orlando. But I never stopped.

I'm not sure I was even competition for myself this time, but today, it was more than enough.

As my legs came to a rest a smile slowly spread across my face. A woman wrapped me in silver foil and a man put a medal around my neck.

You'll never know how much I've earned this medal.

It was as if he read my mind. He pulled me into a hug and then looked into my eyes.

"Congratulations."

"Thank you," I said, grasping the medal as though I'd won the Olympics.

I was pushed into a sea of runners looking for family and friends. The crowds were enormous. The sun was bright and I was starting to feel my aching body. You tend to tune all that out while you're running. Endorphins are a beautiful thing.

Tim was nowhere to be seen.

I finally climbed on top of a barrel where I knew if I couldn't see him, he would eventually see me.

After about thirty minutes scanning every head in the crowd I spotted him.

"Where the hell have you been," I said as he made his way toward me.

"Searching everywhere for you," he said, looking relieved.

A 29-year-old woman had died just after crossing the finish line, and all Tim could think about was all the antibiotics and decongestants I had to consume just to be out there.

He'd been bouncing around between the finish line, the medical tents and the family waiting area, wanting to see me finish, yet concerned I may have had problems.

"And I had just seen this guy in a Winnie the Pooh costume cross the line looking pretty bad. I was hoping you were already in and I just missed you."

"You are kidding me, THAT guy finished ahead of me? Geez."

Tim just stood there staring at me, grinning.

"Come get me down from here," I ordered. "I'm so stiff now I can hardly move."

Tim lifted me to the ground.

"You did it, darlin'," he said squeezing me. "I'm proud of you."

"So what beer are you on?" I said.

"I finished in 3:36."

"So I'm guessing about number four."

"No, I waited for you."

"For an hour and a half? Now that's love."

We asked a fellow runner to take our picture and then we ambled our way back to the hotel where we toasted the day together.

"Want to come back and do it again next year?" Tim asked.

"Absolutely," I said. "Lord willin' and the creek don't rise."

I love running. It makes me feel alive. I guess on some level I also figure as long as I keep running, cancer can't catch me. It's a ridiculous notion, I know. But it helps me to overcome the fear of that rising creek in my mind.

We stayed in Chicago for a couple of days to enjoy the sights and make up for lost calories. (One of my favorite things about marathons). The town was Cubs crazy, unknowingly on its way to yet another baseball heartbreak.

Buildings were lit up with the Cubs logo. Everyone was flying a Cubs flag, and wearing Cubs stuff. One waitress almost kicked us out of a restaurant when we told her we were from Florida.

"It's OK," I said. "We're not Marlin's fans, we were just here to run the marathon."

"OK then, you can eat."

In the end, the Cubs curse was too strong. A fan reaching for a foul ball snatched defeat from the jaws of victory, tipping it away from the outstretched glove of Moises Alou and virtually sealing the Cubs' fate.

They say you've got to live the blues to sing the blues and Chicago has some of the best.

We ended our trip with a visit to a club called Blue Chicago where Big Time Sarah and the BTS Express felt the pain.

On our way home, our flight from Chicago to Atlanta was horribly late. We found ourselves sprinting through the airport in hopes of making a connection home. You have never seen anything so funny as two post marathon runners trying to sprint. I was actually running faster than Tim at first and as he passed me I noticed he wasn't alone. Flying from the bottom of his shoe was a long stream of toilet paper.

"Now where's my camera when I need it," I laughed.

We got to our flight, just as the plane was boarding.

I couldn't wait to see the kids. Danielle was still in her ballet class when we arrived back at the condo. Drew at football practice.

"It's good to be home," Tim said.

Our old friend the ocean was still there. I breathed in the salt air for a moment, then grabbed the car keys and drove down to Danielle's class. I watched through the window as she laced her point shoes and began her bar exercises.

My daughter is beautiful. She is 11, tall and thin with legs that are already a mile long. Where she got them, I have no clue, but I take credit for them anyway.

I didn't cry once in Chicago. But there standing at the window, watching my daughter I felt the tears spill down my face.

Back at home, we ordered pizza for dinner, just as Drew came bounding in the door with Nancy.

He threw his muddy body into me.

"Mommy you were slow, Tim was fast!"

"Thank you for that analysis Andrew, I missed you too."

"Oh Moooooom."

Drew's bright eyes and his white teeth were about all that stood out from the caked on crud around his face.

"Why don't you grab a shower before dinner?"

"Come on mom, I'm not that dirty."

It's hard to imagine he could have been any dirtier, but I was so glad to see him I didn't care.

"OK, but at least wash up a little, and I don't even want to see your fingernails."

He sped off toward the bathroom.

Later that night I watched my children sleeping. Drew, in his room, no longer in perpetual motion, was in the bottom bed of his bunk. A lump moving rhythmically under a pile of Jaguars covers. Danielle, in hers, nestled in one corner of the bed, spiral curls around her face, cuddling a teddy bear that is her nightly companion. The bear is white, and wears blue pajamas with pink breast cancer ribbons all over. Yet another gift from a caring viewer.

The sight of them sleeping peacefully filled my heart to bursting.

When I was little, I went through a stage when I couldn't imagine peaceful slumber. I was scared to sleep by myself. My mother would have to come lie down next to me until I nodded off.

"I'm afraid something is going to get me," I pleaded. "Please don't leave me alone."

If someone left my closet door open I panicked. This sense that something evil was lurking, waiting to engulf me, was overwhelming.

Having cancer is the closest I've come to feeling that malevolent presence since.

It is a battle of wills to keep it away. Good versus evil. The unconditional love of strangers helps to keep my focus on the light.

My family has to love me. The people who are part of Donna's Journal loved me simply because I needed them to. I've learned so much from them about love.

They have made me a better mother, a better wife, and a better member of the human family.

As I write this, I am approaching one year since the end of my chemotherapy.

Next week, I am scheduled for a simple blood test. As if any blood test for a cancer patient could ever be simple.

My palms will sweat, I'll get that nauseous feeling, and when it's all over I hope I'll be relieved.

I have no idea what the future holds. I'll leave that to God.

What I do know is that whatever happens, the strangers who are my friends will be there, to celebrate with me, to worry with me, to pray for me, to fight beside me, to light my path.

And for that, I am forever grateful.

I will do my very best to pass it on.

EPILOGUE

The Donna Hicken Foundation

Lisa Mosley's Story
by Bridget Willis Spruill

"I tell people, worrying about things that are out of your control, makes you so stressed. I was so stressed that if I had been walking this walk by myself, I probably would have taken my life. I am honest when I say that. It's a hard struggle every day to have cancer, or any kind of illness. I can understand how people can take their own lives if they aren't strong."

Lisa Mosley, 34, wife and mother, has an open face with high cheekbones and clear, glowing skin. When she smiles, her brown eyes are alive and sparkling. Her dark brown hair hangs in cascading ringlets that frame her face. Her voice is deep and full.

"When the doctors told me I had cancer, I was alone. Dr. Shegel came in. She told me that I would need a mastectomy immediately, the pathology test came back showing that the cancer was all through the tissue. Everyone said it was so unusual for me to get breast cancer, because there is no family history of it, out of fifty grandchildren, I'm the first one."

Her doctors advised her to have a double mastectomy. "But my right breast was okay," Lisa thought, "the oncologist said there was a fifty-fifty chance that the other one could contract it as well. If I knew then, what I know now, I would have had the double mastectomy." (Lisa is now undergoing tests of her right breast to determine if cancer is there.)

Through all of this, Lisa's three daughters, Sharika, 17, Ja'Lisa,

14, and Ciara, 12, were a godsend to her. "I was blessed with three good girls, very good girls."

Even though Lisa worked full-time while her husband Greg was away, the bills kept piling up. She got to such a low point that she couldn't open them. "I would just put them in the drawer. I couldn't face them. As long as we had a roof over our head and groceries in the fridge, we could make it I thought." But the pressure was too much.

Family members did what they could to help. Her mother-in-law, Oddessa Batts, was there during her recovery, "I never knew my mother-in-law was going to have to bathe me! She took such good care of me. She would change my bandages and everything. By the time the nurses would come to my room, she had done everything."

Mrs. Batts' help didn't stop there. "I used to have these pity parties, and she would say, 'We're not going to have any pity parties. Let's walk or read scriptures or do something.' She made me get up even when I didn't want to. If it wasn't for her, I probably wouldn't be here." Lisa pauses, "God kept her here long enough to take care of me through my sickness, because a year later she died."

Her aunt Catherine helped financially when she could. "She would give me cards and bless me with $50 inside. Auntie Catherine, she's my everything. When I was growing up, my mom and I would go to her for strength."

Lisa's grandfather, Curtis Smith, would check to see if she was taking her medicine, "He'd say, why aren't you taking your medicine? And I'd tell him I couldn't afford the $50 to $100 co-pay."

With the financial hole she found herself in deepening, and so hard to get out of, she turned to the standard forms of support offered to the community, such as food stamps, AFDC, among others. With these she only found red tape of insurmountable levels. They all needed proof of her situation that was hard to come by, and to be suffering with cancer made it doubly so. Some of the people she came in contact with treated her without respect.

After much effort with other agencies and not knowing where else to turn, Lisa was surprised with a phone call from Catholic Charities. "Somehow they got my name. Maybe a friend gave it to them, I don't know. The only thing I know is that Catholic Charities set me up for an appointment to get financial assistance."

Lisa arrived for her appointment promptly. After the paperwork was completed, she began the interview process. "The young lady that helped me was so nice. She asked what kind of treatments I was having and stuff like that."

At first it seemed like another roadblock to Lisa, for a moment she felt she wouldn't be getting the help she needed.

"I told her how hard it was to get anywhere with the other agencies. And that coming from a two income household to a one income household made me so stressed. I told her my doctor said stress will kill you faster than the cancer.

"We got to talking and she said, 'you know what? There is a new charity helping women with breast cancer that is affiliated with Catholic Charities.' And then she told me about the Donna Hicken Foundation. She said, 'I'm going to have someone from the Donna Hicken Foundation call you before 24 hours.' She took all my information down. That was a Thursday and somebody called me on Friday. They set me up for an appointment on Monday."

"My mom, Sharon Carter, went with me to the appointment. We met Julie and Celeste and a lady named Susan. Susan is a cancer survivor and she's traveling all over the world and having chemo, and I'm like, 'you go girl.' They were all so positive. They asked me what I needed, you know, what was on my plate at the time?"

Many of the agencies Lisa sought help from consider a car and a phone to be a luxury. But with children and a job these are necessary. When the DHF helped Lisa she was so shocked because they made it so easy for her.

"They cut through all the red tape. They paid my phone bill and my JEA bill. The Foundation put money towards my rent and paid my car insurance. And they paid my ticket. Now what charity is going to pay a ticket? They put me back on top and brought all my bills current. The Foundation really blessed me financially.

"I hope people will donate to the Donna Hicken Foundation, you know, every penny counts. I want people to know what a relief they were for me. Worrying about your finances is a burden, you feel like you're probably better off dead than alive, 'cause you sit around and worry about your sickness, your bills, your children.

"When you look at someone you never know what they are going through. I always try to be nice to people because you never know. I may look good on the outside, but underneath all this, you see scars. And these scars are here for life. But they make me stronger. And people would never know it looking at me. You know, I try to be right by life and to myself.

"I just want to be at peace. I mean, I'm blessed just to be here. My hope is to stay positive, to stay focused. And I want my daughters not to have to go through what I went through. I just want to be happy. You know, happy with my husband and my children. That's all."

*   *   *

In the few short months since The Donna Hicken Foundation began we have helped dozens of First Coast women like Lisa Mosley with everything from their mortgages to their medications. We've paid their electric bills and their co-pays. We've made sure they have food for their kids and help on days they can't do it all alone.

Catholic Charities has been the partner I knew it would be. Completely yet lovingly screening each recipient to ensure that we are good stewards of people's donations.

Celeste Beale, our treasurer, is our insurance toward that end. Our voice of reason.

"Don't spend it all in one place."

Julie Gillespie, God love her, is still working as a volunteer director. I think she spends more time with tissues at her desk than I ever have. (And trust me that's saying something.)

The three of us have long strategy sessions at the office (Panera Bread). We pore over the numbers and divide up the week's work.

Every now and then one of us, or all of us, depending on who has PMS, will throw up our hands in frustration, only to be handed a fresh miracle and a renewed spirit.

My friend and fellow cancer survivor, Susan Mehrlust is a walking miracle every day. She still must take chemo almost continuously, but it never sinks her. She spends hours with our recipients, on the phone, at the bedside, or in the hospital making sure no one feels alone. Most importantly, she believes they can make it. After all she's living proof.

For all of her years of living with metastatic breast cancer, she still believes it can't get her. Before every check-up, or blood test, or PET scan, she tells me "I still don't think I have cancer."

She says it with a huge smile and you know, I think her body is listening.

Sadly there are still many women whose bodies don't.

They don't respond to the chemo, or their cancer has gone too far by the time it's detected.

One of those women was Shirlene Roberts. The first one of our recipients to lose her battle with breast cancer.

In pictures Shirlene was a healthy glamorous looking African American woman with a smile that I could only describe as stunning. She was 39, and a mother of four. Shirlene fought as hard as she could. But she had a handicap. Early on, she let the fear of knowing, rob her of the chance to save her life. She waited to get a firm diagnosis. Like so many women she hoped that what she didn't know wouldn't hurt her.

One of her sisters would later tell me if Shirlene could leave one message, it would be "DON"T WAIT! Know your body. Get checked. Live!"

By chance, or by divine providence, I had the opportunity to meet Shirlene days before her death. It was just before Christmas.

A lovely, generous woman named Norma Jean May persuaded her colleagues at BellSouth to donate Christmas presents for all of our recipients and their children. Not just any presents, but each child's own wish list! Like so many others who get involved, Norma Jean lost a loved one, her niece, Sharon Parker, to breast cancer. She is driven to ease the pain of those still suffering.

On the morning of December 22nd, Norma Jean, Julie, Celeste and I met at a pre-determined spot and the families each sent someone to pick up the gifts. We were all spent. Really tired. It was a busy time and we'd done our share of venting about how we didn't know how we could do all of this, and oh by the way, hold down full-time demanding jobs.

When it was time to go, Shirlene's family hadn't shown. Turns out, they got lost. I put the gifts in my car and headed for Shirlene's house. To be honest, the idea scared me a little. I knew Shirlene was in tough shape. I wasn't anxious to come face to face with what this disease, my disease, could do. Celeste knew this about me and offered to go instead. For some reason I felt compelled to go. I hope it was mostly out of compassion, but I was curious too. Does that sound morbid? Scared, yet definitely curious.

When I arrived at the house, a small girl, who looked to be about my son's age was in the driveway. Shirlene's daughter. She is a beautiful child with big brown eyes and dark hair, tied in a high pony tail. I had to pry a smile from my hard-wired jaw. We exchanged hellos and then some of Shirlene's other family members appeared at the door ready to help me carry everything inside.

"How is she?" I asked.

A dumb question for sure, but I was struggling.

"She doesn't have long," someone said. "She'd love to see you."

When I walked into her room, Shirlene was curled up in the bed, terribly thin and frail. She looked almost like a sleeping child. Maybe 65 or 70 pounds. But when I entered her field of vision her eyes lit up and that stunning smile spread across her still very pretty face. Her body had been decimated, but her spirit was fully intact.

I held her and kissed her warm cheek and wished I could save her.

"What can I do?" I asked. I felt horribly helpless.

"It's going to be okay," she said consoling me.

"I'm ready and God is ready for me. And Donna, I want you to know," she said, still smiling, "how much peace your Foundation has given me."

Here's this young woman, way too young for this. And there isn't a shred of fear in her. Instead she's telling me she is grateful.

"I can never thank you enough," she said. "Now at least my children won't be left with bills on top of grief."

"You got everything on the wish list?" she had asked me wide-eyed that day we met. "Even the Barbie Jeep?"

"Everything," I said feeling elated at the joy the word brought to her face.

"I can't wait to see my daughter's face."

And she did. Her child's excitement was one of the last things she experienced on this earth.

Shirlene died that weekend, after a beautiful gift-filled morning with her children.

I called Celeste crying.

"You were meant to go there," she said. And we laughed through our tears about our earlier gripes.

A couple of days after Shirlene's death, I found out more about the extraordinary person she was. Long before she became ill, she had experienced a pain far worse than any cancer could bring. She had lost a daughter seven years earlier in a car accident. The child was crossing the street when a motorist hit her. Shirlene and her husband decided, through their grief, to donate their daughter's organs so that she might live on in others. Because of their unselfishness, four children are alive today, including one who has their child's heart.

I believe Shirlene Roberts' heart is still alive as well.

Shirlene fought the good fight and left behind a legacy of love. I'm so grateful the Foundation played a small role in that legacy. It tells me we are moving in the right direction.

When we first started DHF that direction was in question.

We debated how we should go about fundraising. Should we

save until we can endow the effort so we don't have to worry about running out of money, or should we spend it as we get it and trust that people will be generous? We decided on the latter, because there are women who need us now.

Not later.

Later we will have a cure. Now, we need to care for those who are suffering.

We have yet to turn one truly needy woman away. Whenever we start to worry about the bottom line, someone will make a donation. It's uncanny.

Sometimes it's almost to the penny of what we need. The day we wrote a one thousand dollar check as a deposit for Shirlene's funeral, Julie went to the mailbox to find a five-hundred dollar check and two others for $250 each. No notes, no stated reason, just the checks.

And we even built hope a home. Literally. A local builder, Paul Axtell from Classic American Homes, called me one day. "I lost my dear friend Sherri Quist to breast cancer and I want to do something in her memory," he said. "Something that will help women here in our community."

Boy did he help. Paul donated a piece of land and his sub-contractors donated labor and materials. Everyone gave their time and we built a house. It sold before it was even finished to Kathy and Sheldon Levine and the Foundation got a big fat check for $60,000. All that money goes to help First Coast women with breast cancer. WOW! It will come as no surprise when I tell you that Paul is a client of Cynthia Montello.

And as you saw at the front of this book, my friends at Closet Books are donating all the net proceeds from the sale of "The Good Fight" to the Foundation as well.

So buy early and often!

Doors and hearts continue to fly open.